SCISSORS AND COMB
HAIRCUTTING

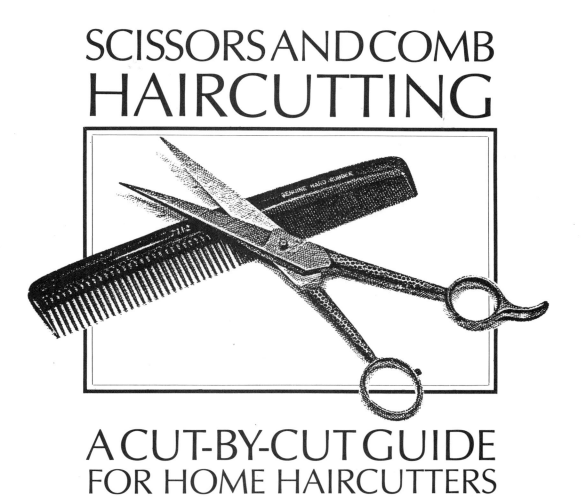

A CUT-BY-CUT GUIDE
FOR HOME HAIRCUTTERS

WRITTEN AND ILLUSTRATED BY
BOB OHNSTAD

You Can Publishing
P.O. Box 11400
Minneapolis, Minnesota 55411
www.howtocuthair.com

00 01 02 03 04 BAN 9 8 7 6 5

Printed in the United States of America

Library of Congress Cataloging in Public Data

Ohnstad, Bob., 1941 -
   Scissors and comb haircutting.

   Includes index.
   1. Haircutting.   I. Title.
TT970.037   1985   646.7'242   84-90072
ISBN 0-916819-01-9 (soft)

Published by
You Can Publishing
P.O. Box 11400
Minneapolis, Minnesota 55411
www.howtocuthair.com

CONTENTS

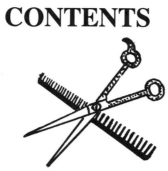

PREFACE

Welcome to the craft of haircutting. You'll find this skilled activity
has abundant benefits: for you there is the satisfaction of producing
something practical and unique with your hands; for the receivers of your
haircuts, the hair's health and appearance is considerably
enhanced, plus there's even a significant contribution to mental
health—a precision-cut head of hair that requires no more than a few
minutes of attention a day encourages a little brighter outlook.

Here you learn how to cut hair, long or short, so your efforts
result in hair that stays in shape all the time, even if windblown,
massaged or handcombed. To make hair so carefree, all you do is follow
the cut-by-cut haircut directions and teach your haircuttees about the
need for a shampoo and towel-drying every day or two. This book proves
there is **BEAUTY IN SIMPLICITY** when it comes to hair.

To introduce myself, I'll begin by explaining how this book came to
be. Before August 20, 1978, the thought of writing a book had never
seriously crossed my mind. On that day, as I lie in a hospital bed
waiting for the results from tests and X-rays, I pondered: What is the
best thing I can do with the limited time I have left? Because
twenty years before I had a kind of lymph gland cancer that is
supposed to recur despite being arrested, I had good reason to expect
the worst verdict on my ailing lung.

I soon learned my illness was pneumonia, but before I was told
that, I decided to write a book that makes available the knowledge
I've gained during my professional career. My question was answered
almost as soon as it came to mind—it came from this background:

● The success I have had in making people happy with their hair.
● Experiences I've had teaching haircutting to friends and relatives.
● A commitment to the notion of self-reliance: my life has been made
simpler and more satisfying because of do-it-myself activities.

I could have written a shorter, more bare-bones book, but I chose
not to for two reasons. First, I wanted to pass along as much hair
knowledge as I could—you always learn best by doing, but if you use
what my experience has taught me, many pitfalls and disappointments
will be avoided. Second, I learn best by knowing the reasons—the
WHY?—behind the subject: I assume the same holds true for you.

In the spirit of WHY?, it's only fair that you know about my basic
values. This book instructs you in **one** of the many ways to cut and
care for hair—my beliefs have limited impact on my haircutting
methods, but the haircare I teach has a number of parts where my
convictions come to the surface. So there is no misunderstanding,
these are the major things I try to keep in mind.

0 0 0

I subscribe to the view of our human condition given by Thomas
Aquinas: we all live in **two different worlds** at the same time—a
spiritual world and a material world. While you can't see or touch the
things that make up the spiritual world, those things are a very real
part of our existence. Included in this unseen world are notions like
values, faith, understanding, feelings of love and compassion—not
much to get your hands on here, but much of a person's time can be
spent dealing with these matters. The material world consists of all
the tangible things: Mother Earth, food, cars, money, homes, a fur
coat, hair, your body—the list of touchables goes on and on.

Aquinas tells us we have a teeter-totter relationship between these
two worlds. The more you live in the material world, the less you can

partake of the spiritual world—on the other hand, the more you are concerned with things of a spiritual nature, the less materialistic your approach to life will be.

As I have tried to fit this dominant belief into my profession, I have learned a simple approach to cutting and caring for hair that results in a pleasing appearance, as well as making it **healthy** and **ignorable**. I give ''ignorable'' haircuts because I want to make it a little easier for my customers to concern themselves with things higher than the hair on their head. Vanity, extra time, concern, and costly resource use can be heaped onto my carefree haircuts, but it's soon obvious the extras are not needed. The **way** the hair is cut insures a good appearance with the least maintenance and concern.

0 0 0

I don't like greed. In the first years of my career, the professional haircare business was a fairly ethical exchange of money for service; since the late 1960s, I've seen it become one of the greediest personal-service businesses. There are many pleasant exceptions to the greedy pro, but money-grubbers abound. Many franchise shops, and even one-location shops, have adopted a quota system: primary importance isn't placed on employees taking care of their customers' needs by cutting hair well—if they don't sell enough extra services and expensive products, they are looking for a new job! The sales motto is: if customers don't spend it here, they will spend it someplace else, so **get** them for all you can! Those with a ''big I—little u'' mentality have taken a service that can be extra positive and made it into something that treats people as little more than objects.

There is ample selfishness and greed in all areas of human affairs; I would like to have a small impact on this part of it.

0 0 0

I believe in stewardship to Mother Earth. Our garden of life must support those who come after us—we have to give the newcomers a fair chance to be all that they can become, instead of having to deal with life-destroying garbage made by us.

I know what we do to hair has minimum impact on acid rain, smog, and the Love Canals we've created. But how we deal with hair is **one** small contribution to these larger problems that is easily avoided when this book's haircare how-to is put into practice.

If you're uncomfortable with the values that shape me, don't put the book down yet. My purpose isn't about preaching these beliefs; the purpose is to clearly show how to give the kinds of precision haircuts most people prefer. My convictions do come out in the haircare parts of the book, and the suggestions for determining the right length make the haircare easy; but the haircutting procedure I teach is a result of over two decades of hands-on experience. Taken as a whole, the book makes possible the less-is-better haircare I advocate, but the hair can be fussed-over as much as you want—THE CHOICE IS YOURS!

* * *

The most beautiful things in life are felt by the heart and not seen by the eyes.
                                                            Helen Keller
There is sufficiency in the world for man's need but not for man's greed.
                                                            Mohandis Gandhi
Our ideals, laws and customs should be based on the proposition that each generation in turn becomes the custodian rather than the absolute owner of our resources—and each generation has the obligation to pass this inheritance on to the future.
                                                            Alden Whitman

HOW TO USE THIS BOOK

This book teaches how to give the kind of precision haircuts that make people **happy** with their hair. To achieve this level of success on your first haircut, and with every haircut you give, the book should be used the way it was intended.

● Get the general idea. Read through the entire book once or twice to get a good overview of the haircutting process—the skills involved and how to go about them. Chapters 9 and 10 should be skimmed: the how-to in these two advanced haircut chapters is much easier to follow when you have experience with the beginner's haircut shown in chapter 8.

● Develop your skills. The most efficient way to use the tools is described along with a simpler, less skilled approach. Either way needs some practice before you can be comfortable with the tools.

● Take care. Pay close attention to the various safety considerations that haircutting requires. The subject index shows all the references to this important matter.

● Last minute review. Before each of your first few haircuts, start with the Overview chapter and read through the chapter on the haircut you will be giving.

● Make it easy on yourself. When you use proper tools, set up the best possible work environment and choose the right persons for your initial haircuts, you go a long ways toward insuring success.

● Let the book guide you. When it comes time to give a haircut, follow the cut-by-cut photos and how-to instructions. Here the book is used as you would a new cookbook: follow it closely to get a good start— when you're comfortable with the basics, you'll be in good shape for experimenting.

● Use the book as a consultant. Solving hair problems, answering questions and dealing with hair myths are important parts of successful haircutting. Refer to the book as needed.

Take care of this book and it will serve the hair needs of future generations. Your children and grand-children will find these basic ways to cut hair as worthwhile and contemporary as you will.

* * *

The best effect of any book is that it excites the reader to self activity. Thomas Carlyle
To read without reflecting is like eating without digesting. Edmund Burke
A good teacher is one who makes himself progressively unnecessary.
Anonymous

1   ABOUT HAIR

1.1 CLOSE-UP OF A HAIR

One of the astonishing things in our world is the snowflake; zillions of those little frozen crystals and each is a one-of-a-kind creation. Despite the uniqueness of snowflakes, there are basic similarities among them. So it is with heads of hair: no two are exactly alike, but there are many similarities from one to the next.

    This first section's examination of hair is concerned with things that are common to all hairs; later sections of this chapter examine the different qualities that make every head of hair unique. To begin, there are four terms used to describe a hair from tip to tip.

A. Four Parts of a Hair

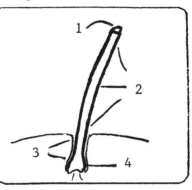

1. End: the oldest part of the hair.
2. Hairshaft: the visible part of a hair.
3. Root: the part of the hair that exists below the skin.
4. Bulb: the little bump found at the bottom of a growing hair. This newest part of the hair is hard to see, but your finger tips can feel it when a hair falls or is pulled out.

The root and bulb are parts of a hair not seen while hair is growing; they are surrounded by the complex growth "factory" we examine next.

B. The Follicle
My dictionary defines a hair follicle as the sheath that surrounds the lower, subcutaneous part of the hair. (It is supposed to be a good dictionary, but that definition doesn't say much about the busy nature of a follicle.)

My description is more detailed: a follicle is that part of the skin surrounding the hair root and bulb, and it produces the different cells that make up a growing hair. The follicle is about 1/4 inch deep, and it has these various parts.

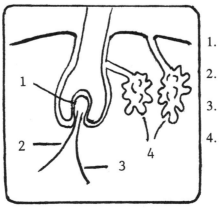

1. Papilla: the site of hair cell production.
2. Blood vessel: the nourishment supplier.
3. Nerve supply: the regulator.
4. Sebaceous glands: the producer of natural oil.

The small cone-shaped elevation at the bottom of the hair follicle is the **papilla**. With its blood and nerve supply, the papilla manufactures the cells that make a growing hair. The papilla is the source of pain you feel when a hair is pulled out prematurely—the bulb grows around the papilla and tugs at it when a hair receives pull-out pressure. The **nerve supply** sends the papilla's pain message to the brain, but more important, it acts as an on/off switch to control the different stages of hairgrowth (described later in this chapter). The **blood vessel** brings the nutrients needed to keep the papilla humming along with its cell-production activities. The **sebaceous glands** produce a natural oil called sebum. This oil travels from the gland, through the duct to the hair root or up to the scalp; eventually it coats all the hair as it journeys on the outside of the hairshafts to the hair ends. Sebaceous glands don't produce much until puberty, and their production slows after age 45–50.

C. The Different Layers of a Hair

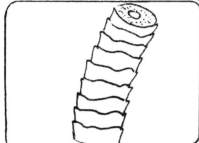 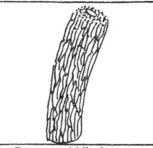 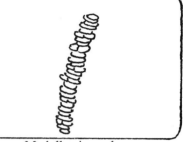

Cuticle: outside layer.   Cortex: middle layer.   Medulla: inner layer.

Depending on how thin or thick a hair is, it has two or three layers. Each hair has a **cuticle** layer composed of hard, round, tubular cells. These outside armor cells protect the softer, inner layers. If the hair is in a healthy condition the cuticle cells lie flat and overlap each other. In this state, the outside layer can perform its primary function of protection, but there is also the added gain of a healthy sheen.

If the cuticle layer becomes damaged the overlapping part of the cell will curl up. This condition diffuses light and the hair appears dull. When the cuticle gets to this state, the soft cortex layer is exposed and damage such as split ends and hair breakage is likely.

The **cortex** layer is made up of long, spindle-shaped cells that lie parallel to the hairshaft's length. These soft cells contain melanin, the color-giving pigment. Melanin combines with air bubbles in the cortex layer to give hair its many shades of brown, blond, black, and red (melanin is absent in gray and white hair).

The third layer of cells—which may not exist on small diameter hair—is the **medulla.** This inner-most layer is composed of soft, coin-shaped cells stacked on top of each other in a irregular manner.

D. Chemical Composition of Hair

Hair is composed of keratin, a protein substance also found in the skin, finger nails, and toe nails. The approximate chemical make-up of hair is: 50% carbon, 20% oxygen, 20% nitrogen, 5% sulfur, and 5% hydrogen. Because of the nitrogen content of hair, it is a welcome (but slow to decompose) addition to the compost pile or garden.

E. Hair's Function

Those hairs on your head are not there just to be an adornment or a nuisance that must be endured. They function as a little extra cushion against blows to that delicate brain and as an effective temperature insulator. In winter, a large part of a person's body heat is lost through the top of the head; a bald head loses body heat much faster than a full head of hair. In the warm months, hair serves to insulate against the heat of the sun. Other things being equal, a bald person will suffer a heat stroke sooner than a person with abundant hair.

1.2 NUMBER OF HAIRS AND RATE OF GROWTH

The number of hairs on a head and the growth rate are two hair factors that help make every head of hair unique. An average adult head has 120 square inches of hair growing surface (the scalp) with a little less than 1,000 hairs per square inch. Hair color makes a difference: blonds average 120,000 hairs on their heads; brown and black-haired folks, 110,000 hairs; and redheads, 95,000. There are countless exceptions to these averages, but these numbers hold fairly true.

The number of active hair follicles on our heads slowly decreases throughout the course of living, and males have more of a decrease than females. Whereas deer grow new hair follicles throughout their lives, we have to be satisfied with the follicles we are born with.

How fast the hair grows has a relationship to the diameter and color of the hair. Finer, lighter colored hair usually grows 3/8 inch a month. For the rest of us, those hairs can sprout as much as 3/4 inch, however the average is 1/2 inch per month. Darker hair usually grows faster than lighter, coarser hair faster than finer. Gray hairs seem to flourish a little faster than the hair they replace.

The growth rate is the same for each of those 100,000 thread-like objects on the head. While the rate may speed up for gray hairs and it's usually slower for children in their first year or two, the rate otherwise remains constant throughout our lifespan.

1.3 HAIR TYPES

Hair type is another factor that contributes to the uniqueness of every head of hair. The last chapter describes how this subject gets a little muddled by some hair conditions, but for now we'll examine the four general categories used to describe this characteristic of hair.

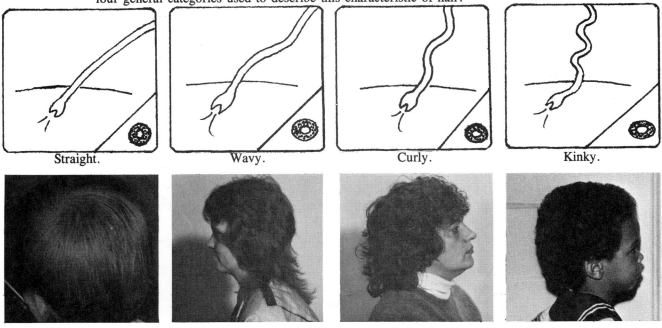

Straight.   Wavy.   Curly.   Kinky.

These drawings and photographs illustrate the differences between the various types of hair. The cross sections of hair, (in the lower right hand corners of the drawings) show straight hair is the roundest and kinky hair is the flattest. Note that the curlier hair is, the more it grows straight **up and out** from the scalp, whereas straighter hair grows out at less of an angle and lies closer to the head. This angle of growth from the scalp leads us to the next subject.

1.4 HAIRGRAIN

From my experience I have found that only a minority of professionals and virtually no customers are aware that every head of hair has a unique **hairgrain.** You need a thorough understanding of hairgrain because this factor determines the lying direction of straighter types of hair; as a result, hairgrain makes a major contribution to the final appearance of your haircuts. In addition, the hairgrain has an impact on the way you use the tools during the haircutting process.

This hair phenomena, sometimes called the hair-growth pattern, has to do with the **direction** the hair grows from the head, and the fact that an individual hair grows out from the scalp in the same general direction as its neighbors.

Hair doesn't grow out from the head in a willy-nilly manner. 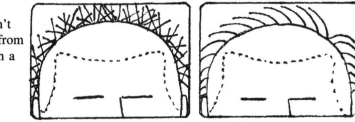 Hair has a fairly uniform way of growing from the head that reflects its hairgrain.

A. My Best Hairgrain Explanation

When I explain hairgrain to my customers, I use the example of a dog with short straight hair. Run your hand through the hair on its back from tail to head: the hair stands on end for a moment, then lies down again, returning to its natural lying position. The hair lies in this particular way because a dog's coat has a definite **hairgrain pattern**: The angle the hairs grow out from the skin is quite uniform from one hair to the next, and it results in the hair having a natural lying position toward the tail.

We humans share this characteristic with our canine friends. Whether it's the tresses on our head, beard hair, or other body hair, there is a definite pattern to the direction hair grows from the skin. While there are gradual changes in the hair's lying direction—and occasionally there are fairly abrupt changes—individual hairs grow out from the skin in the same direction as their next-door neighbors.

If hair grew straight up, the concept of hairgrain would not exist. 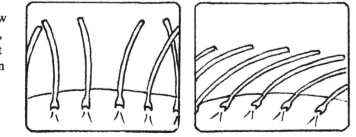 Hair emerges at an angle, with its neighbors having the same angle. Hence, the pattern is created.

B. Two Basic Types of Hairgrain

Every head of hair has its own unique grain—its way of growing out of the scalp. Despite this uniqueness, you will find that there are **two** basic hairgrain patterns that describe nearly all heads of hair.

● **Type 1 hairgrain**: the side hair grows toward the bottom.

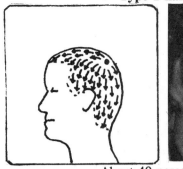 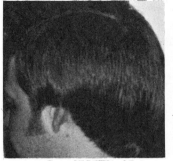 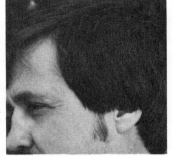 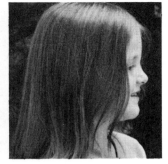

About 40 percent of the people in the world have this type of hair grain. Normally, this hairgrain is found on straight-haired folks.

● **Type 2 hairgrain**: the side hair grows toward the back.

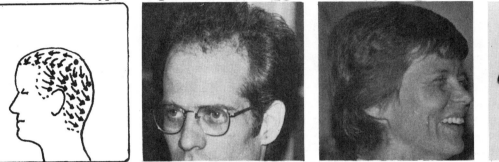 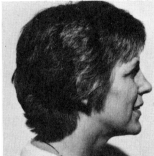

This pattern occurs with the other 60 percent of the world's population. Type 2 hairgrain is usually associated with wavier, curly and kinky hair. (These percentages reflect the part of the world I've worked in—if I were a haircutter in Asia or Africa, the percentages I suggest would be different to some extent.)

A common feature of the Type 2 hairgrain is the ducktail neckline. With a Type 1 grain the hair at the neck normally grows straight down, while a Type 2 usually grows in a pattern of curves and whorls at the nape of the neck—quite like a duck's tail.

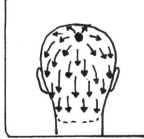 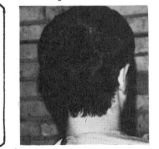 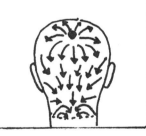 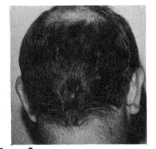

Type 1.   Type 2.

There are many variations of the ducktail neckline; the one shown here is fairly typical (see page 97 for more examples).

C. The Cowlick

Our discussion of the hairgrain now goes to the heart of the matter—the **cowlick**. Despite popular opinion, the cowlick is much more than an ornery tuft of hair that some people have to put up with. To begin unraveling this subject, you should know that **every** person's crown region (the upper back part of the head) has **one** cowlick, and on rare heads you'll find two back there—you may even discover an extra cowlick at or near the front top hairline. This hairgrain phenomena is the starting point that establishes the pattern of the hairgrain; put another way, the cowlick is the **center** of the hairgrain.

When I point out this fact of hair for my customers, I usually describe the cowlick as if it were the axle of a bicycle wheel: the hair in the immediate vicinity is like the spokes of the wheel—they all go out and away from the axle.

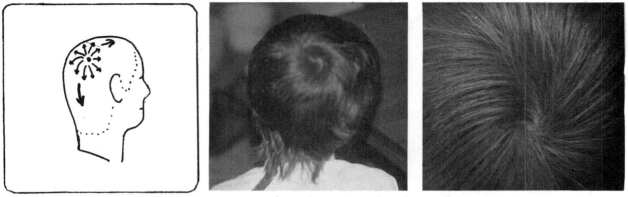

The hair grows away from the center point, the cowlick.

Wherever you find the cowlick in the crown region (in the center area or off-center, toward the front or in a lower position), the hair grows out and away from it: **down** toward the bottom of the neck, and **forward** toward the front of the top of the head. It is **always** the case that the hairgrain is directed toward the front on top, however there are slightly different growth patterns that depend on where the cowlick is positioned. If the cowlick is on the left, you usually find this hairgrain pattern:

Left-side cowlick and its normal hairgrain.

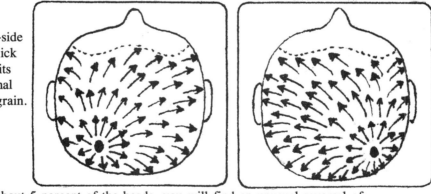

A right-side cowlick usually has this hairgrain pattern.

On about 5 percent of the heads, you will find an unusual reversal of the pattern.

Left-side cowlick with reversed hairgrain.

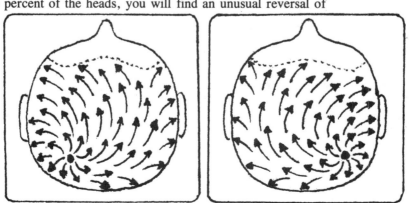

Right-side cowlick with this unusual hairgrain.

When the cowlick is located in the center of the crown region, three different hairgrain patterns are possible:

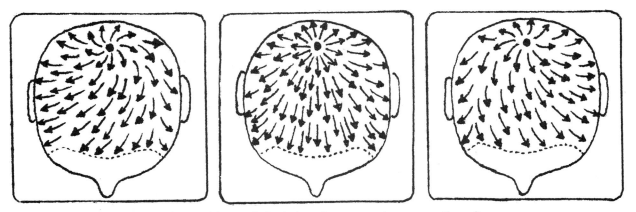

The cowlick's position and the hairgrain pattern that comes from it, contributes to the uniqueness of every head of hair.

D. Cowlick Confusion

How can **every** head of hair have at least one cowlick, yet this fact is known by only a small minority of people? The reason behind this befuddled state has to do with how different lengths and hairtypes are able to **hide** this hairgrain phenomena.

● **Long hair.** Although straight hair is the hairtype most affected by hairgrain and the cowlick, longer straight hair gets heavy and bends downward because of its excess weight and the force of gravity. Because this bending happens near the roots, it's common for the cowlick region to be covered over by long, bent hairs. When this same hair is cut on the shorter side, the surplus weight is gone and the bending no longer occurs—the hair lies the way it wants to and the cowlick can easily be seen.

● **Curly and kinky hair.** These types of hair confuse us because they grow **out** from the scalp like coiled springs:

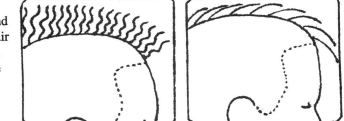

Curly and kinky hair coils out from the head.

In contrast, straighter hair lies close to the head.

Straight (lie down) hair shows more of the hairshaft which makes it easy to see the hair's grain and cowlick. Curlier hair results in a head of hair where all you can see is the hair's ends—the hairgrain and cowlick is well camouflaged.

Curly or kinky types of hair have to be cut quite short to see the hairgrain and cowlick.

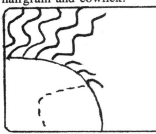

When curly/kinky hair is cut to a length of 1 inch or less (so the first upward bend is cut off), the hairgrain and cowlick shows itself. Once the hair has grown another 1/2 inch, it bends again and springs out from the scalp—the cowlick is back in a state of hiding.

The curlier the hair is, the shorter it must be cut to see the cowlick. This rule also applies if the hairgrain is to have any impact on the hair's lying direction; however, unlike straight hair, this impact is slight because curlier hair can usually be combed or brushed so it lies in any direction when it's cut short.

You will learn in the chapter 7, that wavy, curly, and kinky hairtypes can be cut to just about any length. Straighter kinds of hair tend to have one best length.

E. The Stand-Up Cowlick Problem

Sometimes the hairgrain and cowlick hide. Occasionally the hairgrain's center point makes itself most visible: I am talking about that stubborn tuft of hair that stands out from the rest of the hairs in the crown region. This wild hair problem **only** happens with straight or slightly wavy hair. The curlier types of hair grow **out** from the scalp all over the head, so all of the hair ends blend together—they all stand up, so there can't be any crown region hairs that stand out from the rest.

There are four possible causes for cowlick hairs standing on end, but two or more of these causes may combine to make a little tuft into a major eruption. We begin with the most common source of the problem.

● **Wrong combing direction.** Whenever hair that wants to lie away from the cowlick is combed or brushed in a direction against the natural lying inclination of the hair, you will have stand-up problems. Most commonly this occurs with the hair that grows from the crown area cowlick toward the top front hairline: when the hair is allowed to lie the way it wants to, there is **no** stand-up problem.

<table>
<tr>
<td>Hair is combed with the grain, toward the front.</td>
<td>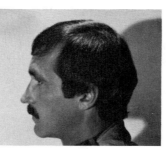</td>
<td>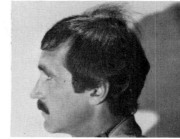</td>
<td>Hair is combed toward the back, which is against the grain.</td>
</tr>
</table>

When you start fighting your hair's natural way of lying, you'll always have stand-up problems.

● **Twin cowlicks.** Less than 10 percent of people exhibit the hairgrain phenomena known as twin or double cowlicks. Two center points in the crown region doesn't always mean the hair sticks out, but on about one-quarter of these folks the hair **between** the cowlicks will want to stand on end, particularily if it is cut too short. The rule is: the closer together twin cowlicks occur, the more the hair growing between the cowlicks will want to stand on end. The consequence of this rule is that you have to leave the hair **longer** so that it will bend and lie down with the other hairs around it.

<table>
<tr>
<td>The hair wants to stand out at the clash-point between the cowlicks.</td>
<td>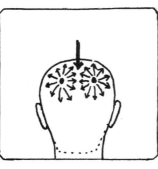</td>
<td>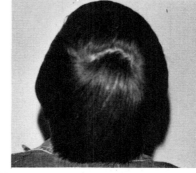</td>
<td>The line you see between the two cowlicks is a natural parting of the hair created by a separation of the hairs that lie toward the front of head and and those lying toward the neck.</td>
</tr>
</table>

● **Low cowlick**. Every head has a cowlick in the crown area, but some rare heads have their cowlick in a lower than normal position.

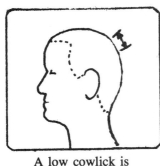
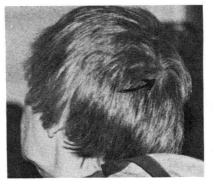
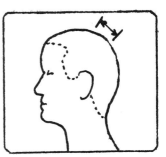

A low cowlick is situated in this area.

Cowlicks are usually found in this area.

The low cowlick produces a stand-out problem because the hair that wants to lie toward the top front of the head has an uphill battle with the forces of gravity.

The arrows point to the uphill area where the hair wants to lie toward the front of the head.

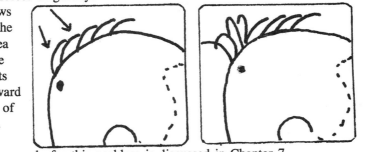

But gravity pulls that hair down, toward the back of the head—when hair doesn't lie the way it wants, stand-out hair is the rule.

The easy remedy for this problem is discussed in Chapter 7.

● **Cut too short.** Fewer than 5 percent of people have a single cowlick in the crown region that has to be left on the longer side. With these folks you find that your best estimate for hair length on top of the head results in the top hair lying well, **but** you end up with a few hairs standing on end in the cowlick area. This rare problem proves cutting hair is not always 100% predictable: you may be a bit off on your length calculations when you encounter a stubborn cowlick like this—just leave it longer the next time you cut it.

F. The Exceptional Hairgrain

Nine times out of ten, the hairgrain on one side of the head is a mirror image of the hairgrain on the other side. Occasionally it's slightly different, however, one head in a hundred will differ a lot: you may find one side growing straight down, while the other side grows toward the back of the head.

The center of the hairgrain is a fairly routine matter, but recently I came across a first: a fellow I was giving a haircut to surprised me with his two extra cowlicks—each was a little more than an inch up from the neck's bottom hairline, about two inches apart, and the "knowledge bump" (located where the spine meets the skull) was directly between them. I've seen a few people with an extra cowlick at the bottom edge of the neck's hairline, but never a cowlick so high up into the back hair—then to see a pair of them! What next?

The "snowflake" nature of hair keeps this an always interesting, sometimes surprising craft. Just when you think you've seen it all, you encounter a head of hair that proves you wrong.

G. Checking the Hairgrain

To determine if you are dealing with a Type 1 or Type 2 hairgrain, comb through the hair and look closely at the direction of the hair coming out of the scalp.

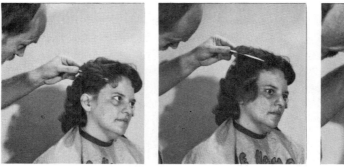

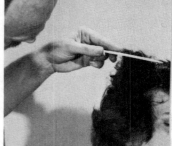

Comb through the hair in an upward direction on the sides and look closely at the base of the hairs that fall from the comb as it moves up up through the hair.

Note the direction of the first 1/2 inch of hair coming out of the follicles: that part of the hair is most influenced by the hairgrain. Longer hair bends downward because of weight and gravity—if you look at the hair beyond the 1/2 inch point, you are likely to see bent hair that gives a false reading.

Use this same upward combing and close inspection to check the back hair for a ducktail neckline. On the top of the head, comb in a front to back direction to check for cowlick(s) and for the direction (to the left or right) that the top wants to lie.

Straighter hair shows its hairgrain at a longer distance from the follicle than do curlier varieties. This means you need to look extra close at the newest part of the hairshafts on wavier and curlier hair.

H. Hairgrain and Genetics

In my first years of barbering my services were limited to men and boys. Since I started giving haircuts to all the members of the family, I have a better picture of the influence genetics has on a person's hair. With this experience I feel safe in saying the hairgrain (as well as all the other major hair characteristics a person has) is determined by genes. The genetic influence is quite noticeable in any family, but it's especially obvious in the identical twins I have for customers. Sometimes the genetic source of a person's hair characteristics is from grand-parents or even great grand-parents, but most often the source is Mom or Dad.

I. Beardgrain

Because there is a section in the last chapter on beard trimming, the grain of the beard needs some attention too.

These are the three general patterns:

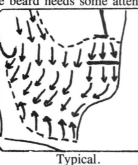

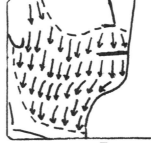

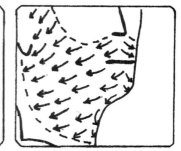

Typical.   Two common exceptions.

The rule is: whiskers generally grow downward except on the lower 1/2 - 2/3 of the neck where the hairs grow upward, and then off to the sides of the neck. There are two exceptions: (1) the neck hair grows down with no upward or reverse grain (2) the hair grows somewhat downward, but mainly toward the sides of the neck.

Men who shave with a safety razor or the old-time straight-edge razor usually have some notion of the beard's grain. If their shaving blade is directed against the grain of the beard, they will get a very close—sometimes too close—shave that can leave the skin irritated and even cause ingrown hairs, infections, and rashes. On the other hand, if the cutting edge travels with the direction of the grain, the result is a less close, but more comfortable shave.

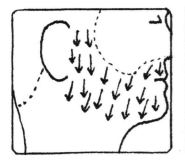

Typical grain on the side of face.

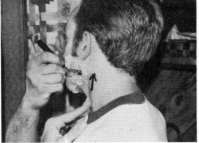

If the blade travels up, it's an extra close shave.

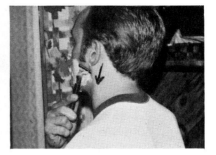

When blade moves down, it's a less close shave.

J. Hairgrain Highpoints

● **Unique, yet similar**. While the hairgrain contributes to a head of hair's uniqueness, nearly everyone's hair can be classified as having a Type 1 or Type 2 hairgrain.

● **Permanent**. The grain of the hair is something a person is born with. It is as unchangeable as fingerprints.

● **The hairgrain is boss**. The grain of the hair determines the lying direction of straight or slightly wavy hair. This natural force on the hair diminishes when the hair is longer than 2 1/2 – 3 inches: then the hair can bend, and its weight plus gravity will have an impact on its lying direction.

● **Curly hair characteristics**. It is difficult to see the hairgrain on wavier and curlier hair because they grow out from the scalp. This hair is less affected by the hairgrain because it can usually lie in any direction, if it's cut short enough. Longer lengths on curlier hair finds it returning to its stand-out-from-the-head nature.

● **The hairgrain's center point**. Everyone has a cowlick in the crown region of their head. Some stand up, but this usually results from not letting the hair around the cowlick lie the way it wants.

1.5 TEXTURE OF HAIR

The texture of the hair refers to the thickness or thinness of individual hairs. The diameter of the hairs on the head can be as large as 1/100 inch or as small as 1/500 inch. For purposes of classification, the terms fine, medium, and coarse are used. Fine hair tends to be lighter in color; coarse hair generally has a darker color. Medium-textured hair can be any color.

Assume that each of these hairs is two inches long.

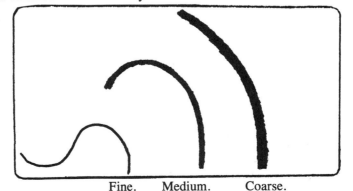

Fine.   Medium.   Coarse.

As this drawing indicates, fine hair is the softest, most bendable of the three.

As chapter 7 points out, texture is the major factor in deciding what is the best length to leave straighter types of hair.

Age has an impact on the hair's diameter. At birth we have the finest-textured hair; by the time we are in puberty the hairs have expanded to their maximum diameter; and when hair turns gray, silver, or white, it's common for it to come in with a coarser texture.

The whole head of hair can be referred to as thick or thin. When hair is described this way, we are **not** talking about the hair's texture, it's a matter of the number of hairs per square inch.

1.6 HAIR GROWTH

A. The Three Stage Cycle

Most people are not aware that their hair maintains a steady process of growth, shedding, and new growth. Many folks believe that when a hair falls out, it's gone forever and they are one step closer to baldness. This notion is at least a mile off the mark! A hair's life cycle has three different stages to go through.

First is the **anagen** stage or the growth part of the cycle. A hair grows at a continuous rate for as little as two years for some people, to as long as six years or more for others. How long a person's hair remains in its growing stage depends on age and genetics: (1) as a teenager you experience a longer anagen stage than you do in your later years (2) the genes your parents passed onto you make all the difference between a short growing season and a long one.

With the second part of the cycle, the **catagen** stage, the papilla stops its production of hair cells. This shutting down stage lasts for 2 – 3 weeks and results in a shrinking of the follicle.

The next step in the cycle is the **telogen** stage. In this part of the process the hair growth factory rests. When the follicle has stopped shrinking, the mature hair hangs around for another 2 – 3 months. During this time the shrunken follicle holds onto the hair unless it is dislodged by shampooing or brushing. At the end of this stage the follicle resumes its normal shape and it's time for another anagen stage; the papilla activates again, and a new hair starts to grow. At this point the old hair either falls out or is pulled out, or the newly emerging hair actually pushes out the old hair. In a couple of weeks the new hair appears from the growth factory and you'll have a happy growing hair for another 2 – 6 years.

At any point in time, over 85 percent your hairs are in the long-lasting anagen stage of the growth cycle—the remainder of the hairs on your head are in either the catogen or telogen stages. This continuous cycle results in a daily shedding of about 50 – 200 hairs. You'll always lose hair. The key to having a healthy growing head of hair is to replace the bailed-out hairs with new ones—to keep that anagen stage coming back for more.

B. Long Versus Short Growing Heads of Hair

Two different people let their hair grow for five years without any haircutting: one ends up with waist-length or longer hair, while the other's locks only grow to about six inches below the neck. This difference is caused by the rate of hairgrowth per month and the length of the anagen or growth part of the cycle.

Eventually a head of hair reaches the point at which it won't get any longer. This does not mean the overall head of hair stops growing (remember, over 85 percent of your hairs are growing all the time). It does mean the oldest, longest hairs on the head have finally reached the catagen stage, soon to be followed by the telogen, the resting and fallout stage. These longest hairs that eventually fallout are continuously being replaced by other long hairs that are approaching the end of their growth cycle. The length of the bottom edge remains constant, but the big majority of hairs continue growing.

1.7 HAIRLOSS

The three stages of hair growth result in a daily shedding of about 50 – 200 hairs. If the daily discard exceeds this amount in a big way, then something out of the ordinary is probably happening. A number of causes create the abnormal loss of hair—some are permanent, some are temporary, and some are not what they appear to be.

A. Confusion About Hairloss
Some of the things we do to our hair results in what **appears** to be excessive hairloss:
● **Hair breakage.** Some folks, especially those with fine-textured hair, suffer hair damage that results in hair breaking off. There are a number of ways to break hair, but chemical processing (permanents, hair straightners) and a lot of swimming in chlorinated water are the two main culprits. You can easily determine breakage by examining bailed-out hairs that come from shampooing or brushing. If these hairs don't have a "bump" on one end (a hair bulb), the hair has broken off. If you can feel the bulb, some other cause is behind the hairloss.
● **Infrequent shampooing.** If people shampoo once a week, they will find much more hair in the tub or sink than if they shampooed daily. Shampooing and brushing, you'll recall, dislodge hairs that are in the telogen stage. If these hairs are not dislodged, eventually they fall out or are pushed out by new growth. If you shampoo weekly, you will have 168 hours of telogen stage hairs waiting to be dislodged, while daily shampooing produces only 24 hours of this natural shedding. Infrequent shampooing makes it appear as if you are losing a lot of hair, but really you're not—unless that scalp gets to the "crusty" stage described in sub-section C-2 on the next page.

B. Temporary Hairloss: Six Possibilities
Anyone can experience extraordinary hairloss in a fairly short period of time. There are a number of possible reasons and dealing with any of them always takes **patience** before the normal growth cycle resumes and the lost hairs are replaced. The different causes are:
● **Physical stress.** Severe fever, major surgery, shock, etc.
● **Emotional stress.** War has done it to many—any extra stressful way of living can do it.
● **Blessed event.** With all the hormonal changes that happen just after childbirth, significant hairloss is almost always experienced.
● **Drugs.** Cortisones and amphetamines will do it. It's also common to lose hair after stopping the use of birth control pills.
● **Hormonal disorders.** Particularly those associated with the thyroid and sex glands.
● **Diet deficiencies.** Without protein the follicles go on vacation. Even vitamin or mineral deficiencies can have a limited impact.

* * *

If we are really being observed by people from outer space, why don't we hear them giggling?   Orben

C. **Permanent Hairloss: The Causes**

When an individual hair follicle permanently stops production, the shut-down is a result of inherited tendencies, or it is caused by something you do or don't do to your hair.

1. **Genetic heritage.**

Your genetic heritage is, by far, the most important factor in permanent hairloss. When it is genetically the right time for that growth factory to shut down, that's exactly what happens despite your best efforts to the contrary—it's all beyond your control.

This shutting down of hair follicles is tied to your hormonal system: at a genetically-determined moment the male hormone, testosterone, accumulates in the blood vessel going to the papilla, shutting it down permanently. The only things that stop this process for men (it's called male-pattern baldness) are castration or taking large doses of the female hormone, estrogen. Ignoring the first possibility, the second possibility works but it has the side effects of breast and hip growth, and facial hairloss.

Permanent hairloss in women is also associated with the male hormone; however, because a woman's hormonal system produces only 25 percent of the testosterone that a man's system does, she loses much less hair than he. In both cases, it's the testosterone that does it. For women, hairloss of this type usually occurs during menopause. At that time the estrogen production slows down, but the testosterone level remains constant, producing limited hairloss. Estrogen hormone therapy may be considered as a solution for women, but there are risks involved, including the possibility of blood clotting and cancer.

2. **Abuse**

People permanently lose their hair when the time has come. However, there are things we can do (or not do) to speed up the process.

● **Crusty scalp**. The next chapter goes into more detail on what happens to the growth factories when you don't shampoo often enough. For now it is enough to say that an accumulation of dandruff, oil, and dirt can produce a covering on the scalp that literally strangles the follicles (and it is so easy to avoid).

● **Hair bending**. When you put constant pressure on those delicate hair follicles, you are asking for big trouble. Many pony-tail wearers have discovered their tightly pulled-back hair has left them with some bald patches. This way of wearing the hair is especially damaging to people with a Type 1 hairgrain: this type of hair wants to lie downward on the sides—pulling the hair back bends the hair near the root, putting much more stress on the hair follicles than would occur with a Type 2 hairgrain. The technical name for this hairloss condition is traction alopecia. While usually a temporary hairloss condition, it can be permanent; at any rate, this approach to wearing the hair makes life miserable for the growth factories—avoid it!

Another, more common example of straining the follicles occurs with people who try to make their hair lie in a direction that's not in harmony with the hairgrain. Combing or brushing the hair against the grain doesn't cause much follicle stress on wavy or curlier types of hair because they grow up and out from the scalp; straighter hair, on the other hand, receives quite a bit of bending near the follicle when the hair isn't lying the way it wants to. While this type of bending is not as severe as you'll have with a pony-tail, I've seen so many people with thinned-out hair where the hair is severely bent for a long period of time, I have to believe traction alopecia has been at work. This rule is a result of my 20+ years of observations: the more hair bends near the root, the more stress on the follicle; the longer this condition occurs, the greater chance of early hairloss.

You can fight that hairgrain until the hair falls out. On the other hand, you can accept what your genes have given you and get a precision haircut that results in the hair lying the way **it** wants to—life with your hair will be much easier and you'll make the most of your hair's health in the process.

3. **Malnutrition of the follicles.**

● **Nutrients**. When the body is deprived of its basic needs, hair is an early casualty. We start with the crucial one.

● Protein. If you've ever seen malnourished people, you know how important protein is to hair: without it there is major hairloss (but who cares about hair when starvation is an everyday concern). Hairloss from this source can be temporary, but it soon becomes permanent.

● Minerals. Iron increases the amount of oxygen in the blood which is important for the growing health of the hair. Weak, easy to damage hair may reflect a deficiency in the needed trace mineral zinc.

● Vitamins. Vitamin E is excellent for the whole circulatory system, so it is important for those follicles and their blood supply. Vitamin C creates a healthy skin and scalp. B vitamins are necessary for normal hairgrowth.

These essential ingredients to healthy hair can be supplemented in pill form, but the best way is to have a wholesome, well-rounded diet.

● **Promoting an extra blood supply**. This is a controversial subject. Many medical experts conclude (based on the amount of blood they see during hair transplant operations) that the heart does a more than adequate job of pumping blood to the top of the head. They would have you believe neither scalp massage nor any other kind of scalp stimulation benefits the growing health of hair—it gets all the blood it needs. I don't agree. Here is the way I (and others) see it:

● Given the forces of gravity, the top of the head is the place on the body that tends to get short-changed when it comes to the blood supply—this is the only part of the head that experiences hairloss.

● When blood circulation to the extremities (feet, lower legs, hands) diminishes, the shorter hairs that grow there quit growing—without enough blood, the hair factories shut down.

● A scalp massage turns a cool, pale-white scalp to a warm, pink state that comes from increased blood flow. If nothing else, the increased blood flow brings an extra supply of nutrients—a little added treat for those top hair follicles. It sure can't do any harm.

You won't alter the genetic program in store for your hair, but until **proven** wrong, I'll continue to believe you help prevent premature hairloss by promoting an extra supply of blood to the top of the dome. Stand on your head if you want, but at least give yourself an occasional scalp massage.

1.8 MYTHS ABOUT HAIR

I doubt there is anything in this world surrounded by more utter nonsense than hair. In my years of haircutting I've heard the full range of tales and legends, quick-fix remedies, and screw-ball reasons for hair doing the things it does. Knowledge of this wide world of hokum is important to you because a large part of what people do—or don't do—to their hair is based on these hair-brained ideas.

Our wide world of hair mythology begins with the one that is probably the most widely held.

A. Hair Fashion

There is no myth about the existence of hair fashions, but there is a
big myth about its application. We see in the mass-media or among our
friends and acquaintances (who have probably been influenced by the
media) someone with a becoming hairstyle, and we think that's for me!
The problem with this keep-up-with-the-Joneses approach, is that
rarely will a person who wants a certain look to their hair have the
right kind of hair for that look. Hair variables such as the
grain, texture, and the type of hair are **crucial** to the hair's
appearance. You can give the best, most appropriate kind of haircut
for the look a person has in mind, but if they have the **wrong** hair
for that look, you'll have a long-faced haircuttee on your hands!

A classic example of this folly occurred in the 1970s and 1980s
with the feathered-back hairstyles. Farrah Fawcett popularized it and
suddenly they were lined-up to get it. I think these styles, with the
sides lying toward the back of the head and the bangs mainly off the
forehead, are a big improvement over the bangs-on-the-forehead styles
of the 1960s (the forehead is oily enough without any help from hair
lying on it—a good way to promote acne problems). Despite the
advantages there are problems when you strive for hair like Farrah's.

Farrah has a thick head of hair and it's slightly wavy with a Type
2 hairgrain. For those of us with a Type 1 hairgrain, our hair needs
bending devices and/or a body-wave permanent to achieve what Farrah
manages without much effort. Besides the natural state of her hair,
Farrah, like others who appear before the camera, has a hair stylist
to get her hair just right before onstage appearances: a half-hour or
more has been spent fussing over those locks before you see her. Great
for her, but who has the time or abilities to do it for themself?

The endless parade of new hairstyles in the past 10 – 15 years has
added momentum to the hair fashion myth. The ''latest thing'' comes into
being to satisfy the needs of a small percentage of people, with the
hope that it might catch on with a much wider population. Those who
seek these creations are, for the most part, the easily bored (another
term for a type of depression) and those trying to find some sort of
quick-fix for their ego problems. The creators of these styles (the
stylist and often a sponsoring manufacturer or distributor of hair
products) make sure their hair-dos need much more than just a new kind
of haircut: costly extras (products, bending appliances, permanents,
haircoloring etc.,) **must** be used to achieve the desired look.

Playing the hair fashion game is a losing game. Occasionally you'll
conform to the latest; most of the time you end up with a style not
suited to your hair—unless you get into expensive (and damaging) ways
of changing the natural state of your hair. Lots of money, frustration
and concern is expended in a game where the rules keep changing and
damaged hair is the usual outcome. Many have played this no-win game
so long, they don't know what it is to have a healthy head of hair.

B. Training Hair

The myth that hair will do whatever we want must be laid to rest.
Wishful thinking has it that by continuously combing and brushing the
hair in the direction you want it to lie, you eventually **change**
the hair's preferred way of lying. As I have pointed out, the

* * *

When all think alike, no one thinks very much.   Walter Lippmann
We forfeit three-fourths of ourselves in order to be like other
people.   Arthur Shopenhauer

hairgrain is completely unchangeable: when you train hair you simply grow it long enough so it **bends** into your idea of how it should lie. This is a problem that grows on you: longer hair is heavy hair, longer heavy hair is a mop that wants to flop around. To keep that hair under control you must use hairspray or hairdressing and keep combing it and combing it. To top it off, those bent hairs are happy to bail-out before their time (traction alopecia wins again).

A common example of this myth has to do with the American male and the left-side part. For unknown reasons it became the custom for males to part their hair on the left side of the head, with the top hair combed over toward the right side, and the upper-back hair combed over the crown region and down the back of the head. If you have straighter hair this way to wear the hair works well **only if** the hairgrain goes that way. If the hairgrain dictates a right-side part, a life-long battle occurs—the hair (and perhaps a little mental health) is the loser. Chapter 6, section 12 shows how to part hair.

Another example of training in action occurs with men who try to comb all of the top and upper side hair straight back. This way of wearing the hair, called a pompadour, became popular decades ago; but you **must** have wavy hair (or curly hair cut quite short) if the top hair is to lie toward the back easily. Straight hair combs back on top **only if** it's quite long so it can bend back away from its forward, natural lying preferences. With straight hair, the comb-it-back training battle begins with the kind of stand-up problems discussed back on page 8. In time the hair gets long enough to lie down, but by then you have a heavy mop that's always a struggle to keep in place— especially when freshly shampooed. Besides a messy head of hair, that poor dome is full of bent hairs and stressed follicles.

C. **Hair Grows Faster In Some Areas of the Head**

Scalp hairs in the anagen stage are all growing out at the same rate. This uniform growth rate may include a few hairs growing a tad slower or faster than the rest, but this difference is so small it couldn't be seen. The popularity of this myth comes from a couple of sources:

● Assume you have given an excellent haircut that has every hair lying perfect. If the person has a Type 2 hairgrain and a ducktail neckline, they'll find the hair stands out from the head around the bottom of the sides and back as it grows longer. This flippy hair is caused by excess length and weight that makes the hair bend **downward** from the forces of gravity, rather than lying with the hairgrain toward the back on the sides, and in toward the ducktail at the back of the head—whenever hair doesn't lie the way it wants, flippy, stand-out hair is the result. At the same time, the hair on the upper portions of the head lies well: the uninformed person sees that flipping-out hair and thinks it grows faster than the rest of the hair.

● Uneven cutting is another possible cause for this misconception. When the hair is not cut smoothly, you'll have longer hairs that tend to stand out as they grow longer. Again, hairs that stick out from the bulk of the hairs are seen as fast growing hair.

D. **Cutting Causes the Hair to Become Coarser and Grow Faster**

Men in particular love this common belief. We tend to think this way because of changes in male beard growth. When we are young, the beard starts as fine, soft hair (peach fuzz), and, through time and the action of our hormones, it becomes coarse, fast-growing hair. Because that facial hair is shaved many times during this process of change, we assume that shaving **causes** the change. Not true. Facial hair gets a coarser texture and grows faster with or without shaving—changes in hormones during puberty controls the process. Cutting hair does **nothing** to the hair other than make it shorter.

The most common example of this hair myth in action has to do with the excessive eyebrow growth that is common with males over 30 years. Many fellows avoid cutting those long hairs because they think the cutting causes those hairs to grow faster, to become more numerous and coarser. Incorrect! Hormones change short hairs into long ones; there is nothing you can or cannot do to change this fact of middle age.

The same cutting-causes-faster-growth notion spills over the hair on our heads, although here there is an extra factor that contributes to this myth. Yes, hair seems to grow faster after a haircut, but it's really a matter of how hair growth shows itself on different hair lengths. If your hair is 5 – 6 inches long you'll be less aware of your hair's steady growth rate than you would be if your hair is cut to a length of 1 – 2 inches.

E. Straight Hair Grows Faster than Curly Hair

There is no difference in the growth rate among the different types of hair; however, straight hair does show its growth more. This is due to the way straight hair's ends grow straight away from the follicle and scalp. Curly hair, on the other hand, takes a winding path as it grows and this hides the actual growth rate. If a curly-haired person and someone with straight hair both get the same short haircuts, after 3 months of growth their hairs are about 1 1/2 inches long. The first illustration shows the visual difference in growth—the last shows the actual difference when the hairs are stretched out.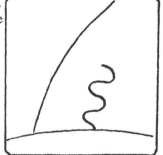

F. Hair Grows Faster in the Summer, Slower in the Winter

Many people are absolutely positive their hair grows faster in the summer, and slower during the cold months. Their reasons are hard to determine, but they stubbornly hang onto this notion. Perhaps they see the vegetable world growing during the warm months and dormant in the cold months, and think hairgrowth works in a similar manner. Their reasoning aside, the fact is, growth rate is as steady as the march of time—neither the temperature nor season of the year has any impact.

One possible explanation for this myth is that people tend to grow their hair longer during the cold months, and wear it shorter during the warm part of the year. In the winter you have a warm, comfortable ally on your head; during the hot weather you have a sweaty burden to deal with. If you feel comfortable with your longer hair, you're less likely to be aware of its growth than when it is shorter (and has to be kept short for comfort's sake). With shorter hair in the summer the rule, we get back to a question of awareness: would you be more aware of your monthly 1/2 inch growth if your hair is cut to a length of 1 – 2 inches, or would you notice it more if it's 6 inches long?

G. Too Much Shampooing Causes Baldness

Wrong! Wrong!! Wrong!!! When you shampoo, you unavoidably remove a large portion of the 100 or so hairs you are bound to shed each day.

Those telogen stage hairs accumulate at the bottom of the sink and it looks like another step toward a shiney scalp (a bigger pile of hair is seen if you don't shampoo often). If you hadn't shampooed, that hair would have been lost in less observable ways: as you brushed or combed, or as a new hair growing beneath the old one pushed it out. The next chapter explains why you have a much better chance to keep your hair growing if you keep that hair and scalp clean.

H. Shampooing Makes the Hair Less Manageable
Natural oil, hairdressing or hairspray have enough weight and sticking power to keep hair held down. Shampooing removes these "restraints" and the hair is free to lie in whatever direction it wants. There are two conditions that don't get along with hair being free to lie the way it wants—these conditions affect any head of hair, but straighter hair has the most problems.

1. **Botched haircut.** When hair is unevenly cut, it must have extra weight or stickiness to keep from showing its chopped-up cutting.

2. **Fighting the hairgrain.** When a person is unaware of, or doesn't respect the natural lying preferences of the hair, heavy holding help is needed to coax those stubborn hairs into their dreams and schemes.

When either or both of these conditions exist, shampooing does make hair less manageable. A person with these conditions usually has to wait 1 – 3 days after a shampoo before their hair doesn't give them a scare when they see a mirror (more time if no hairdressing or spray is used). Because both hairgrain battles and lousy haircuts are optional, this notion of unmanageability from shampooing is another myth.

The precision haircuts you're about to learn makes shampooing simple, even a pleasure. All that's needed is a little acceptance of the hair's natural lying preferences (hairgrain) and unmanageable hair becomes a thing of the past.

I. Different Shampoos are Necessary for Oily, Normal, or Dry Hair
To the contrary, I suggest you avoid brands of shampoo that have a oily, normal, and dry hair version. I've used Nitrazine paper to test the differences between the three versions, and my findings indicate shampoos for oily hair usually have a higher pH than those for dry hair. High pH (high alkaline) shampoos are strong concoctions that will, over a period of time, cause severe hairshaft damage (the next chapter covers hair damage, shampoos and pH in detail).

Perhaps the reason different versions of the same shampoo came into being has to do with a strong shampoo's ability to produce lots of lather—this makes it extra effective in removing oil from the hair.

Another possibility is a strong shampoo's ability to create a roughed-up cuticle layer: this effectively slows the oil's trip to the ends of the hairshafts, but it makes for tangled hair.

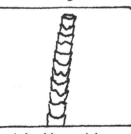 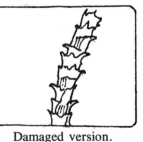

A healthy cuticle.   Damaged version.

There isn't a shampoo made that has any impact on the amount of sebum produced by those sebaceous glands; the aging process, hormones and genetics control the quantity. Most people have to shampoo daily to keep natural oil under control—to shampoo this often without damaging the hair, a low pH shampoo (also called "acid-balanced") must be used.

J. Grow the Hair Long to Cover Up Thinning Hair

Men **cling** to this one; even some women who find their hair
thinning in later life think this is the only way to go. Wrong again.
Because of the extra weight, long hair lies flat on top of the
head, reducing the natural fullness of the hair. When you add to that
the excess oils or hairdressing and spray needed to keep longer hair
from flopping around, the result is starkly thin-looking hair.

Hair in this
condition sticks
together in strands
of 10 – 100 hairs,
revealing a shiney
scalp underneath.
Which do you think
gives better
coverage, . . .

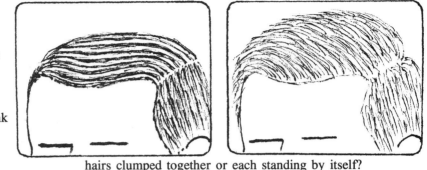

hairs clumped together or each standing by itself?

The best way to handle thinning hair is to cut it short (usually
1 1/2 – 2 inches depending on the fineness or coarseness of the hair).
Then, with a shampoo at least every other day, the hair has body and
appears more full because the hairs don't stick together. These two
fellows consented to having their big "flap" cut off—the hair on top
was 5 – 6 inches long before cutting, and 2 inches after.

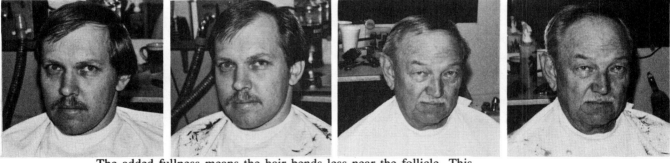

The added fullness means the hair bends less near the follicle. This
shorter length also makes shampooing easy—the clean hair approach
makes the most of what you have while providing maximum growing health
to the survivors. An added bonus comes with windblown hair: the
shorter top eliminates long chunks of hair hanging out here or there.

K. Men and Women Need Different Hair Products

Yes, there are differences between the sexes and their hair. The
balding or thinning process affects men much more than women. Some men
experience a short-growing hair problem around the bottom edges of
their head of hair; a problem not associated with women. Despite these
minor exceptions, no real difference exists between the two sexes in
terms of their hair, and they do not require different procedures or
products to keep their hair healthy. As far as I can tell hair
products labelled for men or women are just Madison Avenue hype.

L. Permanents Create Carefree Hair

Billions of dollars are spent annually by people who are told: If you
want to shampoo and towel-dry your hair, and be able to forget it for
the rest of the day, you need a permanent. Another favorite $ales
approach is built around the permanent's ability to give limp hair
some extra fullness—also called "volume" by the sellers.

The kind of haircuts you learn here proves you don't need a permanent to have low-maintenance hair, and you can get maximum fullness without the expensive treatment. If you want to change your natural hair into something wavy, curly or kinky, a permanent is the answer—but, as the next chapter points out, you pay much more than money for the change.

M. Thinning Shears are the Tool to Use on Thick, Heavy Hair

I'm afraid not. In fact, thinning-out-the-hair is one of the worst things that can be done to any head of hair. When you use thinning shears, the cuts start at about the halfway point on the hairshafts your hand (or comb) is holding. Those toothed cutters take one chomp there, and perhaps another chomp closer to the ends as the hand slides further out on the hairshafts. This process (usually done to the hair on top, sometimes all over) results in some of the hair being quite a bit shorter than the rest.

If you do this to any type hair, especially coarse hair, you get a lot of shorter hairs standing straight on end and pushing out the neighboring, longer hairs.

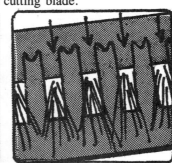

Thinned-out hair.   No thinning.

Besides poor lying hair, thinning shears also damage the hairshafts. To explain this, we need to take a close look at what happens when the blade with 28 (to as many as 46) teeth meets the cutting blade.

Many hairs are held by each small indentation on the top of the teeth—these are the hairs that get cut.

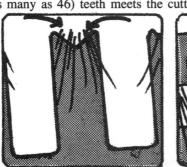

However, more hair slips down between the teeth and remain uncut.

When the cutting blade closes down on the teeth, each indentation holds too much hair. Most hairs gets cut, but some get squeezed off to the edge of the indentation where the hair is **partially cut.** The thinners nick the hairshafts—the result looks like stomped-on straw.

Hair damaged by the use of thinning shears.

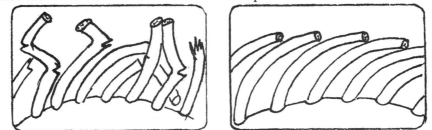

Hair cut by plain scissors.

When a hairshaft is nicked, the soft cortex layer is exposed; this makes the hair very prone to damage such as split ends and breakage.

Folks who have had their hair thinned-out have a hard time with clean hair. Shampooing thinned-out hair removes heavy natural oil (or

* * *

Imagination was given man to compensate him for what he is not. A sense of humor was provided to console him for what he is.

                                                                          Anonymous

You grow up the day you have the first real laugh—at yourself.

                                                                          Ethel Barrymore

whatever else is holding it down), thus freeing those nicked hairs to stand out in all directions. When you add to this a lot of shorter hairs pushing out the longer hairs, a hairy disaster is created until enough natural oil is back on the hair to tame it down.

Using thinning shears is a sloppy, imprecise, and unhealthy way of cutting hair. The best way to handle thick, heavy hair is to cut it as short as possible, particularly on the top, with plain scissors. When you cut off the excess length while leaving the hair just long enough to lie well, you have effectively thinned the hair without using those destructive thinning shears.

N. Razor-Cutting is the Best Way to Cut Hair So It Lies Well

The notion that a better haircut results when you **slice** the ends of hair with a razor sounds very plausible. Advocates will tell you a razor-cut leaves each hair's end slightly tapered so that all the hair lies extra smooth. In fact, you create two hair problems with the sliced approach, and precision haircutting is virtually impossible with the use of a razor.

● Slicing the ends of the hair leaves the cortex layer of the hair much more exposed than it is when cut by scissors. When the soft cortex is exposed, the hair is extra vulnerable to the many ways it can be damaged.

● Razor-cutting results in hair ends that curl up; a close view of hair cut this way reveals a head full of frizzy ends that stand out from the rest of of the hair.

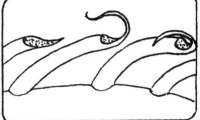

● Success with razor-cutting requires a very stationary head and the **exact** same pushing pressure of the cutting blade against the hair ends, all over the head of hair. With a lot of experience, you may be able to do a good cutting job, however, then you still have the unhealthy consequences shown above.

As in the use of thinning shears, this is an imprecise way to cut that leaves hair sick or, at least, in a damage prone condition. This book teaches how to pull the hair out from the scalp and cut it so as to inflict the least damage on the inner layers—the blunt-cut with scissors is, by far, the healthiest method of cutting hair.

O. If You're Born Without Hair, You'll Go Bald Early

According to this myth: if you are born with a lot hair, you won't go bald; if you come into the world with a hairless scalp, there is no hope for keeping those hairs that eventually do appear. What will be thought of next??

While many bald men have been born with shiny domes, and there are plenty of men who kept a full head of hair who just happened to be born with abundant hair, it is also the case that the opposite conditions occur with equal frequency. This is one more feeble attempt to explain something without knowing the facts.

* * *

Childhood is that wonderful time when all you had to do to lose weight was to take a bath.   Anonymous

Sound travels much slower than light. Some of the things you tell your kids don't reach them until they are in their forties.   Anonymous

Laughter is the shortest distance between two people.   Victor Borge

P. Wash-and-Wear Haircare Requires Too Much Work

Yes, a shampoo and towel-dry every day or two is too much toil **if** the hair is poorly cut, or the hair is long enough to be considered a mop, or the hair must be bent to lie the way you want. These situations make the clean hair approach a drudgery that is not worth the effort.

No, wash-and-wear haircare is not too much work if the hair is given the precision haircuts taught here and you can get along with the natural lie of your hair. In fact, a haircut every couple of months and a 3-minute shampoo and towel-dry every day or two takes much less of your time than any other approach: the haircut insures your hair won't need one more minute of concern during the day. That amounts to 3 minutes out of a day's worth of 1,440 minutes: 3/1,440 of a day to make those hairs ignorable and as healthy as can be!

Q. Hair Keeps Growing After You are Long Gone

Yes, there's even a fairly popular myth about hair and death. This legend has it that a person's hair continues growing after they're gone from this world. I'm afraid not—when your physical plant stops operating, the growth factories also quit. But, hair does **appear** to grow after death because of a limitation in measuring hair's growth. You measure a hair from the skin or scalp to the hair tip. **Yes**, a few days after death, longer hair will protrude from the skin or scalp, but this is a consequence of human physiology. Our bodies are made up of over 90 percent water. When we die, we start dehydrating; that is, we shrink and shrivel because the body's water evaporates. Hair, in contrast, is composed of lifeless cells that don't have any significant moisture content: it does not shrink. As the skin surrounding the hairshaft (the root and the bulb) shrinks inward, the hair remains constant and you end up with a little more distance between the skin and the hair tip. It's the illusion of hair growth, not the reality.

R. You Need Innate Creative Talents to be a Skilled Haircutter

This common myth is promoted by professional haircutters for their own ends. To the ordinary person watching the haircut process, there doesn't seem to be much rhyme or reason to what is going on: a snip here and a snip there, throw in a little fancy tool handling, add a dash of double-talk, show them some decent results while gently extoling your "magic" and you have them hoodwinked into thinking that haircutting is best left to the experts. This mystification of the craft is understandable from the point of view of wanting to preserve one's livelihood—but understandable or not, it's still a myth.

As you read on and put into practice this book's how-to, you will see that haircutting requires no special abilities—you, like millions before you, can learn this enjoyable, worthwhile skill.

I suppose I could fill a book writing about hair mythology, but these are the more common ones, and enough is enough. Let's leave these hair-raising tales and discuss a more positive subject: healthy haircare.

* * *

Nothing in life is to be feared, it is only to be understood.   M. Curie
It's harder to conceal ignorance than to acquire knowledge.   Anonymous
A mistake recognized is half-corrected.   Anonymous
The art of being wise is the art of knowing what to overlook.   W. James

2 HEALTHY HAIRCARE

2.1 HAIRCARE TEACHING

A frustrating thing can happen when you become a haircutter. Let's say you give someone an almost perfect haircut (an extra-precise cutting with the hair at its best length and shape), the kind you feel good about and your haircuttee tells you it's the best they've ever had! All this good stuff and a week later you see that person with their hair looking as if a hurricane had struck! Because of confusion arising from the world of hair myths and a mountain of malarkey created by those who make big money from haircare, people end up doing many unhealthy things to their hair. For you, this means your ability to give precision haircuts is not enough: **you** must spend time educating your haircuttees—you have to become a **teacher**!

You want to make people **happy** with their hair and your cutting efforts. Producing healthy-looking and healthy-growing hair that's simple to care for is a sure path to pleasant results. To reach these goals you have to teach hair facts and myths, and the dos and don'ts.

2.2 THE DOS

The rules to follow for a healthy head of hair are very simple. You will find this approach takes the **least** possible time, money, concern, and resource use, while it **maximizes** the healthy growth and healthy appearance of the hair.

A. Shampoo Daily or at Least Every Other Day
This is the first and most important rule for healthy hair. By keeping hair and scalp clean, you control dandruff, keep a healthy sheen, and the hair maintains a good shape throughout the day. These benefits are easily achieved with a three-minute shampoo and towel-dry.

B. Use the Hands for a Comb
When you teach people to groom their hair by handcombing, you're helping make life a little easier. No longer will they have to be sure their comb or brush is with them at all times, but more important, the old preoccupation with every hair being in place becomes an unnecessary part of the past. Handcombing is relaxed and extra easy, and your comb is always at your fingertips.

C. Give Yourself a Scalp Massage Several Times a Day
A good, vigorous massage turns a pale-white scalp to a warm-pink color by increasing the blood flow to the top of the head. It's a healthy treat for the hair follicles, and it feels good too!

D. **A Haircut Every Two or Three Months**

When you get those old ends cut off and remove hard-to-manage hair length, your efforts result in hair that is healthy and easily maintained. A precision haircut, cut to the right length and shape, is not only the **key** to an easy shampoo, it also keeps the hair well shaped after handcombing or a scalp massage.

E. **Some Problems to Expect with the Dos**

There is nothing complicated or hard to learn about the dos. For many people, simple haircare makes sense—a little sharing of knowledge and they get right into it. For others, your task is to help them **change** haircare habits they have built up over years.

There are many reasons why people don't shampoo very often. The more common ones are fear of hairloss, tangled, painful hair, reluctance to spend time and effort taming the messiness that a shampoo creates (if the hair has been poorly cut), and good old laziness. Whatever the reason, take the time to teach some basic hair knowledge such as: the stages of hair growth and shedding; the need to control dandruff; why hair gets snarled and how to make it healthy. After teaching, get a little pushy—push enough so they give your new approach to haircare a fair try. Yes, old habits are hard to break, but they are soon forgotten—the benefits of this simple, healthy approach are apparent as soon as they are put into practice.

When it comes to handcombing and the occasional scalp massage, it's largely a matter of getting away from the old notion that every hair on the head must be in its never changing place. The I-will-be-in-complete-control-at-all-times approach is a wearisome, usually frustrating way to handle 100,000 hairs. In contrast, a precision-cut hairstyle and a little wash-and-wear haircare gives you hair that fits the head no matter which way it lies. Folks who try out this approach soon see there really isn't anything to be concerned about: whether the hair is windblown, handcombed, or given a scalp massage, the hair goes back to the way it wants to lie and it looks good that way.

To switch from every-hair-in-its-place to this relaxed way of going will be difficult for some. The following photos will help convince the skeptics—each set of photos show handcombed hair, before and after the haircut.

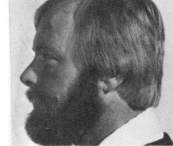

An equal-length cut.

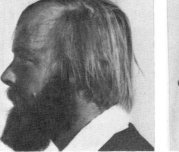

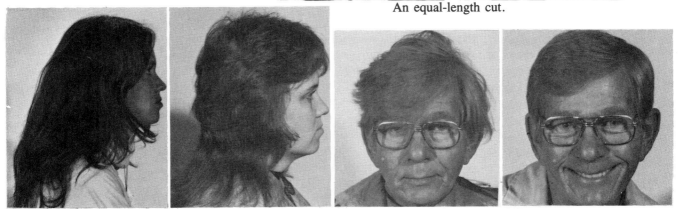

A long, layered cut.   A short, full cut.

2.3 HOW-TO FOR THE DOS

A. The Right Way to Shampoo

Have a regular shampoo schedule. The best way to go is a shampoo and towel-dry every day. Most people find the first thing in the morning is the best time to do it because sleeping usually makes a mess of the hair. If you make it the first task of the day, (it is a refreshing way to get rolling,) the hair is usually air-dried in less than a half-hour. An alternative to the daily shampoo is to do it every other day; again, because sleeping makes the hair flatten down or get flippy, it's a good idea on the mornings you don't shampoo to thoroughly wet your hair with warm water, and then towel-dry as if you had shampooed. Warm water softens the hair and returns it to the natural way it wants to lie.

The goal whenever you shampoo is to do a thorough cleaning job. Getting the hair thoroughly clean means removing **all** the dirt, dandruff and oils that coat the scalp and hairshafts. When the hair is 100% clean, (one or two shampoo applications will usually do it), the hair squeaks as your finger tips grasp and slide out on a group of hairshafts. This is the sound you want to hear on the hair all over your head. Here's how:

1. If you don't shampoo every day, spend a minute massaging your scalp to loosen dirt and dandruff. This can be done by using the pads of your finger tips or a brush with widely-spaced bristles (page 53 shows the preferred type of brush).
2. Wet hair and scalp with warm water and apply a small amount of shampoo to the hands. Mountains of lather are not needed on this first shampoo application—you get that if a second application is given.
3. Rub the shampoo between the hands and distribute it as evenly as possible over the outer layer (ends) of the hair. Using a rotary motion, work the shampoo down to the scalp with finger tips or brush. Give your hair and scalp a fairly vigorous workout, but don't be rough with the hair—wet hair is softened fragile hair, prone to breakage.
4. Rinse thoroughly with warm water. Poor rinsing leaves a film on the hair, preventing it from having any sheen.
5. Time to check for squeaks. If you don't hear that squeaking sound, repeat the shampooing process—one more application ought to do it.
6. Towel-dry. With shorter heads of hair you can give the hair a fairly vigorous towel-drying, but with longer hair, particularily fine hair, you should wrap the towel around the hair and "blot" it as dry as possible. Remember, wet hair is always prone to breakage in its softened condition—longer, fine hair even more so.
7. After you have towel-dried, use a brush with widely-spaced bristles to gently brush the hair in the direction you want it to lie. The hair lies best if this direction goes along with the hair's grain, or only slightly bends away from the grain. Let the hair air-dry and follow up with another brushing. If you are in a hurry for the hair to dry after towel-drying, or you want to add a little extra fullness, the hair can be drum-dried with your fingers (page 85 shows the how-to).

B. Shampooing the Little Ones

Children, from infancy to age four or five, need special handling if they are to grow up with a positive attitude toward shampooing. All the shampoo how-tos apply to the tykes, in addition practice:

● **A gentle touch**. In a child's first year, take extra care to avoid putting pressure on the soft spot on the top of the head.

Children, up to about school age, usually are quite sensitive to **any** kind of pressure on their scalp: go slow and easy with them. Youngsters normally have fine hair that likes to tangle: be sure it's gently, but thoroughly brushed out before shampooing.

● **The recline way to shampoo**. For a child's first four to five years, **you** should shampoo their hair for them using the recline method of shampooing. This is the same method used in barber and beauty shops: the shampooer lays the head back (face to the ceiling) into the shampoo bowl. This can be accomplished at home by using a high stool in front of a sink or by cradling them back in a tub. When a child sits up in a tub or stands in a shower, they always end up with water and shampoo getting in their eyes—no wonder so many children grow up with **contempt** for shampooing.

● **Use low pH shampoo**. It is important to use the mild shampoos recommended later in this chapter. Children's hair is very prone to the kind of damage that results in tangled hair—strong shampoos will always do it. Avoid "baby" shampoos: while they may not sting the eyes, the hair damage I've seen on folks who used this stuff, tells me it ought to be outlawed (it always cleared-up when they switched over to low pH shampoos).

C. **How to Handcomb**

Well, there is not much to it: all you do is use your fingers as if they were the teeth of a comb. Exactly which way you use those pinkies depends on the type of hair you have.

● **Straight and wavy hair**. Use your fingers as you would a comb or brush on these kinds of hair: the fingertips (instead of the teeth or bristles) reach all the way down to the scalp as the groomers move through the hair. The fingers travel in any direction you like, but if you go with the hairgrain, you're assured of hair that lies its best.

With a feathered-back hairstyle, the hands go in a front to back direction. The results come out like this:

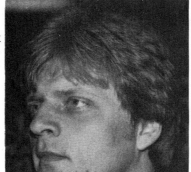

If the top hair wants to go off to one side, a sideways path through the hair gives this appearance.

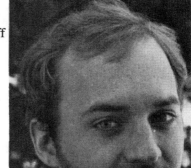

● **The curly and kinky varieties**. Hair that takes a winding path out from the head needs a different approach because it's usually heavy and thick—those blunt fingertips have a hard time moving through the hair.

Use the fingers like a hairpick to make the hair's ends stand out in a smooth shape. To do it, insert your spread-out fingers into the hair and lift out, or grab the hairs between the palm of the hand and the finger tips and pull straight out. The results come out something like this.

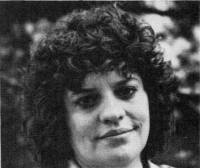

D. **The Invigorating Scalp Massage**

The objective with a scalp massage is to promote an extra supply of

blood to the top of the head. At the least, an increased flow of blood
brings an extra supply of nutrients for the hair follicles, plus, it
does **feel good** to get some stimulation to an area of the body that
doesn't get much. There are a couple of techniques for transforming
that pale-white skin to a warm, healthy pink.

● **The fingertips workout.**

The fingertip pads massage the entire head
vigorously for a couple of minutes. Use a
2 – 3 inch circular motion with firm downward
pressure that **moves** the scalp. You could
also use a brush in the same way.

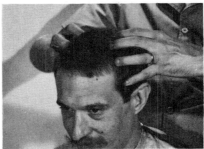

This method works well with shorter hair, and with longer hair if
it is undamaged. With damaged hair you may cause pain and pull out
some hairs—the next approach works best for sick hair.

● **The push-it-to-the-top method.** Here you use your hands in two
different ways.

The insides of the hands
move from the sides to
the top with a firm
pressure. Use this same
technique with one hand
starting at the forehead,
the other at the nape of
the neck.

The spread fingers
technique is used in a
similar way, but here
the fingertip pads are
in contact with the
scalp.

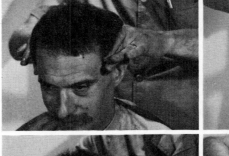

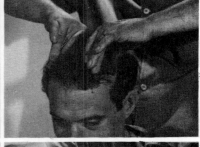

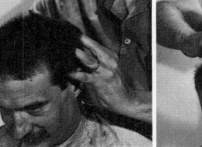

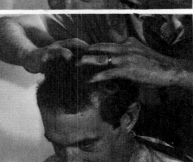

These methods are effective whether doing it to
yourself or to someone else. However, if you
want to increase the effectiveness and add a
whole lot of enjoyment to the massage, use a
vibrator massager like the one shown here. If
you've never had one of these on your head,
you're in for a real treat (great for an aching
neck or back too)!

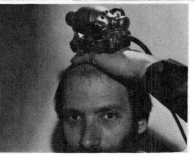

E. A Haircut Every Two or Three Months
The right haircut makes healthy haircare simple, and it's a healthy
thing to do from the standpoint of removing damaged ends. The how-to
for cutting begins after this chapter.

2.4 THE DON'TS

A few folks have strong hair that flourishes no matter what kind of
hurtful things they do to it. Then there are the rest of us who have

to take special care to avoid the many ways hair can be damaged. It ain't fair, but. . . .

Before healthy hair is transformed into a pile of straw, it usually goes through a few worsening stages of damage. To begin, you'll notice a lack of sheen—that dullness is caused by the cuticle layer being roughed-up instead of lying flat. About this time you get into a somewhat painful brushing/combing stage; instead of moving easily through the hair, the groomer has difficulty and the follicles let you know pull-out pressure is being applied. Then the lights go out: instead of a lack of sheen, the hair now becomes totally drab as it absorbs any light that may hit it. At this point the hair is entering the frazzled stage with split ends common and broken hairs showing up in the brush or comb—the hair not only makes others wince when they see it, it's very painful to attempt any kind of haircare.

You get frazzled hair from a variety of causes; however, the worst culprits come from the things we pay money for. Of course there are beneficial products for hair, but many of the items available to consumers must be avoided if we want healthy hair. In the following list, the most common causes of damage come first. Keep in mind that when you have damaged hair, you may have only one basic cause, but most likely you'll have some combination of these causes behind it.

A. **Permanents: Chemical Carnage for Hair**
The first don't is the big one. The permanent wave hoax is a multi-billion dollar a year business that causes more damage to human hair than any other single source.

This hair treatment makes straighter types of hair wavy, curly, even kinky. The hair is rolled up on two-inch-long rods, all over the head, and a high pH chemical solution is applied to alter the way each hair's cells lie alongside each other. After a period of time a neutralizer is applied to stop the chemical action of the first application. How curly the hair gets depends mainly on the size of the rods: if you use large diameter rods, you will have a softer, body-wave curl; the smallest rods produce a tight, kinky curl.

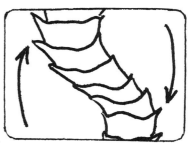

Whatever size rods are used, you'll find after the hair has been treated, individual hairs take on the appearance of a stretched-out spring.

If the hair was given a body-wave perm, the the spring would be stretched out more; a kinky-type perm would be more tightly coiled.

Altering the way hair cells lie alongside each other invites major hairshaft damage. The outside armor cells normally lie smoothly; after a perm, they lie roughly on the outside of the new curves.

At the very least, a permanent roughs up the cuticle layer, leaving the hair so it's easily tangled and prone to the many ways it can be damaged. At its worst, a perm destroys hair by causing major hair breakage. Between these two extremes you can expect dull, sheenless hair, and spit ends are also quite common.

Here are some more things to keep in mind about permanents:

● **How bad will it be**? Permanents have been described as a controlled-damage way to change the natural state of the hair. Being able to "control" this process depends on factors such as the strength and porosity of the hair, how strong the solution is and how long it's left on the hair before neutralizer is applied, the size of the rods (more damage with smaller diameter rods), etc. These different factors make it extremely difficult to really control how much damage is done: it usually takes several permanents before you can zero-in on the right combination that minimizes the damage.

● **The same stuff for different reasons**. Hair straighteners are basically the same concoction as permanents, but as the name suggests, it is used to make the hair straighter. Kinky hair can become curly, sometimes even wavy; curly hair can turn into soft waves. All of the problems associated with permanents are also true for straighteners, but for some reason, hair breakage is much more common.

● **Even the name is a hoax**. The dictionary defines permanent as something that is fixed and lasting—hair "permanents" are neither of these. The curl hair has right after a perm will slowly return to its natural state; the treated hair may not be totally straight again, but it gets much straighter than right after the perm. Permanents are also temporary because only the treated hair curls—all the new growth will be its natural self. A bit of this and a bit of that.

● **The dirty trick about permanents**. Perms are usually sold to folks with straight, fine, limp hair that lies close to the scalp. The sales pitch promises the hair will have added body, fullness, and volume. Yes a permanent does that, but fine hair is the weakest kind and it's most prone to the damage a perm treatment will do. This book teaches how to give straight, small-diameter hair the type of haircuts that maximize the hair's natural body and fullness—you get all the benefits of a perm without any damage.

Now for the other side of the coin. Permanents have been around since the 1920s, and they'll probably keep going strong until head shaving is the norm. While most perms are unnecessary, a few folks have problem heads of hair that can benefit from a perm. A curly perm provides help because curly hair stands out from the head and tends to hide problems, while straighter hair lies down **except** for the problem areas. If a perm is given, these tips minimize the damage:

● Never give a permanent to a head of hair that has any remnants of the last permanent on the hair. Get all of the old permanent cut off before applying the next chemical blast. When you apply a perm to hair with old perm on it, you are asking for double or triple damage. This rule also applies to hair damaged by other means such as harsh shampoos or haircoloring. It takes strong, healthy hair to withstand the damage permanents do.

● If you have a permanent, don't use a hair dryer after a shampoo. Always let the hair air-dry after you blot-dry it with a towel. Never brush out the hair while it is still wet. When it is dry, use a comb or brush with wide-spaced teeth to **gently** untangle the curls.

B. Strong Shampoos

Coming in a close second behind permanents as the biggest cause of hair damage are the high pH shampoos available on drug store shelves.

● **High pH (alkaline) shampoos**. These are mainly old brand-name favorites left over from the 1950s and 60s when most people shampooed once or twice a week at most. Infrequent shampooing means minimum contact with the strong chemicals in those shampoos, and it means you have a large accumulation of natural oil to help protect the hair. (These popular shampoos from the past have an alkaline pH level from 7 to 10 or more on the 1 to 14 pH scale; hair and skin is slightly acidic at a 4.5 to 6.0 level.)

Since the mid-1960s we have been developing frequent shampoo habits; today a majority of people prefer the daily wash-and-wear way to care for hair. There are many benefits to the clean hair approach, but if you use the high pH shampoos from yesteryear, your hair soon gets to the split end and breakage stage.

● **Dandruff shampoos**. To my knowledge, all popular dandruff shampoos are fairly effective in controlling those white flakes, but they're also high pH shampoos that do heavy damage to the hairshafts. Some folks with coarse, strong hair can use these shampoos without doing damage, but for the rest of us, they are bad trouble (page 38 describes a healthier way to handle dandruff).

● **Bar soap**. Some people don't care what they use on their hair, and their hair shows it! Bar soap is almost always highly alkaline, and if used long enough, it makes the hair into a frizz-ball disaster. Hair destruction also occurs if you are careless when washing the face and neck: leave just a little of those soap suds in the hair after washing, and you can expect to have a split-end halo around the edges.

Avoiding hair damage from strong shampoos is very easy—the next section has the recommended mild shampoos.

C. Haircoloring

People in the United States spend over **twenty billion dollars** a year on their hair: the business of changing the hair's color brings in a major chunk of the bucks. Like permanents, this kind of chemical application is damaging to hair at best, totally destructive at worst.

You can tint, frost, rinse, dye, and even bleach those hairs, but when you fiddle with the hair's color the cuticle layer gets damaged. It is common to have dull hair, split ends, hair breakage, even an inflamed scalp (the worst problems occur when peroxide is used).

Recent scientific studies suggest haircoloring preparations are the cause of scalp cancer. Strong chemicals go into haircoloring products; they would seem to be a lot stronger than has been thought.

D. Electrical Appliances

Blow-dryers and curling irons burn the hair, transforming it into a pile of straw. The change is gradual, but over time the hair loses its sheen, develops split ends, and can get to the point of breakage.

The haircuts in this book do lend themselves to the use of any type hair appliance, but excellent, damage-free results come from the recommended towel and air-drying approach.

E. Environmental Factors

If you were careful to avoid the above major causes of hair damage, your hair can still be damaged by the things in our environment.

● **Sun**. Those solar rays, in addition to lightening the color of hair (the summer blond), also dry-out and damage the ends of the hair.

● **Chemicals in water**. I don't know about the other chemicals, but chlorine is very hard on hair. I've seen a number of highschoolers who were on swimming teams: those with finer-textured hair could not grow their hair long—it would break off before reaching a length of two inches. In extreme cases, I've seen blond hair turn a greenish color.

● **Air**. Industrial centers and gas burning vehicles have added together to make our skies unhealthy to those with damage-prone hair.

Environmental sources of damage are hard to avoid, but having the hair cut once every couple of months will remove those over-exposed ends before they get to the frazzled stage.

F. Hairsprays and Dressings

These aids do little damage to the hair, but they create a mental strain that serves no purpose. It's a losing proposition to try to keep those hairs as if they were cast in bronze: a windy day or a little touch causes distress. Seems to me people ought to have better things on their minds than worries about hair being out of place.

G. Problems with the Don'ts

As with the dos of healthy haircare, the don'ts require changes of habits. Most of us have some difficulty with change, but haircare don'ts are extra hard to deal with because of the brainwashing that surrounds hair. To teach about the don'ts, you must stand up to the massive $ales job the media pushes at us daily. When you consider that the average 18 year-old has been bombarded by over one-half million T.V. commercials, a mass-media outlook on hair and its care forms at a very young age. (Added to this is over 40 viewing-hours a week—the people seen on T.V. always spend time with a hairstylist just before you see them—the message about how hair should be may not be direct, but it is there.) As if media indoctrination wasn't enough, there are plenty of greedy professionals who push their patrons into buying any and all extras that promise ''beauty and acceptance'. The net result is a lot of people doing foolish, damaging things to their hair, while convinced they're doing the right thing.

In the face of all this misinformation, you come along and propose a natural haircare approach that hardly anyone has heard of: when is the last time you heard or saw an ad for natural haircare? This less-is-better way of caring for hair doesn't bring in the bucks, but there is no doubt that it leaves the hair in the healthiest condition.

Again, it all boils down to being an **educator**. After teaching, push enough so your haircuttees give the simple approach an honest try: they'll soon see what it is to have healthy hair.

2.5 RECOMMENDED COMMERCIAL HAIRCARE PRODUCTS

A. Shampoo

Frequent shampooing requires a mild shampoo. The pH level of these shampoos are in the 4.5 - 6.0 range—the same level as hair and skin.
● **Salon Selectives #5**. This mild shampoo is quite concentrated—a little goes a long way. Our family has used this product for several years and we haven't had a sick hair the whole time (three of the four of us

* * *

The itch for things—so brilliantly injected by those who make the sell them—is in effect a virus draining the soul of contentment. A man never earns enough, a woman is never beautiful enough, clothes are never new enough, the house is never furnished enough, . . . There is a point at which salvation lies in stepping off the escalator, of
saying, "Enough: What I have will do . . ."   Marya Mannes
Let advertisers spend the same amount of money improving their product that they do on advertising and they wouldn't have to advertise it.
                                                             Will Rogers

have fine-textured, easy to damage hair). You can buy this shampoo in a 15 ounce bottle for about $2.00 in any drugstore.

● **Vidal Sassoon Shampoos**. This is similar in quality to Salon Selectives, but it seems to be a little less concentrated and a bit more expensive.

● **Pert Plus**. This inexpensive mild shampoo also has a conditioner in it. The conditioner seems to keep the shampoo from lathering very much, but it does a good job.

I would expect any shampoo that claims to be low pH or acid-balanced is mild enough to be used on a daily basis. From my own experience I can only recommend these three.

On the negative side, each of these shampoos have a long list of ingredients on the back label that only a chemist could pronounce. The homemade shampoos on the next page will get you back to the basics.

B. Conditioners

In the middle 1960s hair conditioners were virtually unheard of. Why do you suppose they have become such a common part of American life? Permanents, haircoloring, strong shampoos and using dryers and curling irons has made them an important pain-saver: conditioners won't mend wrecked hair, but they do coat the hairshafts after shampooing, thus reducing the tangles and snarls that come with abused hair. If people avoided the don'ts and practiced the dos, conditioners would fast become obsolete. Assuming this won't happen, I know those with wrecked heads of hair will get some relief from these hair-coating agents.

● **Salon Selectives Conditioner**. If their conditioner is as good as their shampoo, I would guess this is good stuff. At discount stores it's about $2.50 for 15 ounces.

● **R-K Moisturizing Creme Protein Conditioner**. I have seen this product tame and soften damaged, straw-like hair, but as with all conditioners, there is no lasting benefit: each time the hair is shampooed, conditioner must be used—until the damaged hair is cut off. At barber and beauty shops, 4 ounces cost around $5.00.

These conditioners, like the shampoos, contain exotic chemical ingredients; if you want to avoid unpronounceables, use the lanolin product described in the next section.

Late Addition

The good folks at my neighborhood food co-op tell me "Tom's of Maine" product line includes superb shampoo and conditioner made from all natural ingredients. Their price is a little higher than average, but the ingredients cost more than the unpronounceables put into other commercial products. I haven't run out of my old shampoo yet, but when I do, I'll give it a try (the co-op folks haven't given me a bum steer yet). Tom's products are standard co-op items.

C. Grooming Aids

As you know, I think the old time every-hair-must-be-in-its-place attitude is a needless burden to one's mental health. On the other hand, I know that some folks just can't accept the casual, more relaxed approach I advocate. And then there is that rare one or two percent of the population whose difficult hair can benefit from a little holding help.

● **Dusharme Lanolin Hairdressing**. This is an old time product that comes to us from sheep. It is their natural oil, obtained from boiling their wool. A two-ounce jar sells for less than $2.00 at your local pharmacy; use it sparingly and it will last a long time. It keeps hair soft and bendable, and it gives fly-away hair a little holding power. In addition, lanolin imparts a little extra glossiness that helps to hide the dull look caused by damage to the cuticle layer of the hairs.

To use it, just rub a **tiny** amount between your hands and distribute it evenly over the outer layer of the hair ends after the shampoo and towel-dry. Work it through the hair, then comb or brush and you are set to go.

If you feel the need to use a conditioner, lanolin has the same basic effect as a conditioner, but you don't have to wash 99 percent of it off the hair and down the drain. Just apply a tiny amount after towel-drying—as you brush through the hair you'll find it helps minimize snarls and tangles.

● **R-K Groom And Set**. This product is available at the local barber or beautician. An 8 ounce bottle costs about $4.50 and lasts a long time. Spray it on after the shampoo and towel-dry, then comb or brush the hair the way you want it to lie. When the hair has dried, comb or brush it out again, and you'll have softly held hair you can run your hands through—the hair keeps returning to its set position. R-K makes quality products that perform well, but they are high priced.

2.6 HOMEMADE HAIRCARE

Only in recent times have people accepted the ease and expense of the commercial haircare products. My dear mother is experienced in the homemade approach: she is the source of most of this old time how-to.

A. Homemade Shampoos
● **Dirt-cheap shampoo**. This may be the least expensive shampoo in the world, but it will do a thoroughly adequate job of cleaning the hair and scalp.
● Grate 1 ounce of a bar of a mild soap such as Kirk's Castile.
● Add grated soap to 8 ounces of boiling distilled water and simmer for 5 minutes while stirring occasionally.
● After it has cooled, put it in a bottle and it's ready for use.

Some additions can be made to your home brew. For your sense of smell, add a few drops of essential oil: oil of lemon, wintergreen, or clove are possibilities. Some folks with damage prone hair may find this shampoo needs to be milder. You can lower the pH level by adding juice from a lemon or lime. To get your shampoo to the preferred 4.5 – 6.0 pH level, test it with Nitrazine paper (available at the drug store). This testing paper shows you when you have added enough of the acidic juice. Many different beneficial herbs can be added to the boiling water and then strained off before adding the soap. Jeanne Rose's Herbal Body Book (Grosset & Dunlap, 1976) gives how-to details, and tells which herbs help different hair and scalp problems. It should be available at the library.

● **Egg shampoo**. Mom first used this method back in the 1920s when she was a beautician. This simple approach does an excellent job of cleaning the hair and scalp, and it leaves the hair sparkling. Try it.
● Wash the egg thoroughly, then crack it into a bowl and beat.
● Apply half of this protein treat to your hair and shampoo as if you were using a soap shampoo.
● Rinse out the egg with **luke warm water**—hot water gives you a mess that is similar to the beginning stage of scrambled eggs.
● Repeat the procedure with the rest of the egg.
● For a finishing touch, give the hair a rinse with lemon (see below).

Carla Emery's Old Fashioned Recipe Book (Bantam Books, 1977) offers other good make-it-yourself shampoos.

B. Low pH Rinse

These old-timers effectively lower the pH level of the hair after the shampoo; they also give the hair added sheen.

● **Vinegar rinse**. Add 3 – 4 tablespoons of apple cider vinegar to 2 cups of water.

● **Lemon rinse**. Squeeze half of a lemon into 2 cups of water. Either of these work well, but Mom tells me that the lemon rinse should be used on lighter hair, and the vinegar on darker hair.

To use a rinse, just pour it through the hair after you have shampooed and rinsed with water. Position the head over a large pan and repeat the rinse with what the pan catches. Then finish with a warm water rinsing. After you towel-dry and have brushed, you'll find the rinse helped to minimize snarls. These rinses give off a slight odor until the hair dries; but then it's gone.

C. Hair Conditioning Treatments

● **Mayonnaise treatment**. My nephew's roommate passed this along to me as a sure cure for ailing hair. After a shampoo and towel-dry, head to the refrigerator for the mayo. Distribute a couple of tablespoons of it through the hair, leave it on for two hours, rinse well, and your hair is happy!

● **Hot oil treatment**. This is an old cure-all for ravaged cuticle cells that is still used today, even in the most expensive hair salons. First, thoroughly shampoo and rinse. Next, apply about an ounce of olive oil to the hair. Wrap the hair in one or two steaming hot (but not too hot) towels and place a plastic shower cap over the towels—a plastic bag or Saran Wrap could also be used. Leave it on for ten minutes and then shampoo as usual. You will probably need 2 – 3 applications of shampoo to remove all of the oil.

D. The Patch Test

I have never known anyone to have any problems with the commercial or homemade products recommended here. However, because some people have allergic reactions to certain chemicals, you might want to rub a little of the product you intend to use on the nape of the neck. Place a band-aid over it and leave it on for a day to see if any redness or swelling occurs. Such a reaction tells you not to use the product.

2.7 REMEDIES FOR HAIR AND SCALP PROBLEMS

Some of these subjects have been touched on in earlier parts of the book; any remaining gaps are filled-in here. Before we start, I should emphasize: nearly all these problems wouldn't exist if people observed the dos and don't of healthy haircare.

A. Excessive Oiliness

Many people complain about their oily hair and how it seems worse now than in past years. It's doubtful they are, in fact, experiencing more sebaceous gland production; instead, they are waking up to the steady flow they've had since puberty. Awareness of oil is tied to the way haircare has changed in the last decade or two. In the 1950s and 1960s infrequent shampooing was the rule. Men shampooed once a week or less, then smacked their hair down with hairdressing. On average, women wore their hair longer at that time, and typically gave it a once-a-week shampoo and set, with lots of hairspray to hold it till the next week. The longer styles worn by women plus hairspray, and the greasy stuff fellows used were effective ways to hide the oil accumulation. With the swing to wash-and-wear haircare, the hair lies fine when it's clean; when oil gets out on the hairshafts, it makes the hair lie quite differently. The old haircare masked your awareness of the oil— today's haircare lets you know how productive those little glands are.

Some folks produce more oil than others, but as pointed out in the last chapter, there is no way to regulate this condition. Two things can be done that **seem** to slow down the oil glands: (1) You can damage the hair so the cuticle layer cells curl up, thereby slowing the oil's trip to the ends. (2) You can grow the hair long which means it takes longer for the oil to reach the ends.

The only healthy way to control sebum production is by frequent shampooing with a mild shampoo. Most people have to shampoo daily to keep the oil off the hair—the kind of haircuts taught here make daily shampooing extra easy. Here are a few other things to keep in mind:

● **The right time to shampoo**. When hair is shampooed has an impact on the oily condition. If you shampoo before bedtime, the oil has an eight-hour headstart on the coming day. A morning shampoo prevents the oil showing up on the ends during the middle of the day.

● **Where is that smell coming from?** If a person goes three or four days or more without shampooing, the oil gives off a real strong odor. People with this condition don't seem to be aware of how bad that sebum smells. If someone you know has this problem, you can convince that person about the need to shampoo more often by having them wash their hands and smell them; have them massage their scalp and smell their hands again. The difference in the two smells will prove your point and encourage frequent shampooing.

● **Strange things happen to hair**. Whenever hair gets loaded with oil, the lie of your hair is in for some changes:

● Wild hair. It tends to make a mess of how the hair lies, especially if you have fine-textured hair. These photos, before and after a shampoo, are good testimony.

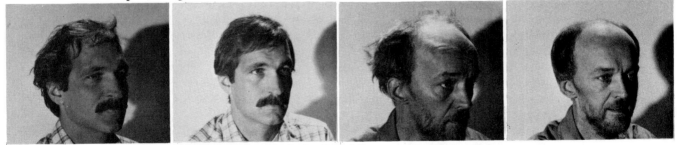

● A hairgrain clash explodes. A ducktail neckline or a double cowlick has a tendency to stand out from the rest of the hair when it's clean—when the oil builds up, the hair pops out.

● Your hairtype appears to change. Straight hair will get wavy, and wavy hair turns curly. The oil makes the hair stick together, multiplying the hair's tendency to wave or curl.

● Thinning hair becomes invisible. Oil is heavy enough to make hair lie flat on the scalp, and it makes the hair clump together into strands of many hairs. Those strands have spaces between them which shows off the scalp—a sure way to achieve bare-minimum coverage.

* * *

Learn to laugh at yourself; you'll never cease to be amused.   Anonymous

B. Hair That Does Not Lie Well

This common complaint results from a number of different causes. Any of the following can create flippy, messy lying hair; when there are two or more of these conditions present, things go from bad to worse.

● **A bad haircut**. There are a lot of haircutters who either don't know how to cut hair evenly or they just don't care. The precision haircuts you are about to learn solves this problem.

● **Damaged hair**. If the cuticle layer is curled up or the ends are split, the hair lies in all sorts of weird directions. Follow the dos and don'ts to a healthy head of hair.

● **Fighting the grain**. When you try to comb or brush straight hair against its natural growth pattern (the hairgrain), or, if you leave the hair so long that it bends away from its natural lying inclinations, you are guaranteed a head of hair that does not lie well. Cut the hair so that it lies the way **it** wants, and don't force it into some contrary position.

● **Thinned-out hair**. Those thinning shears make a disaster out of any head of hair. Cutting hair with plain scissors takes care of this.

● **Clashing hairgrain**. A double cowlick in the crown region or a ducktail neckline (especially if you have coarser textured, straight hair) can result in the hair standing out from the head. Solving this problem requires you to cut the hair to the **right length** (pages 96 – 98 tells all about it).

● **Excessive oiliness**. As the last section pointed out, if natural oil coats the hair, the hair clumps together and refuses to fit the head. Frequent shampooing is the **only** answer.

● **Slept-on hair**. It is a rare person who can sleep a night away and not wake up with hair sticking out in different directions. A morning shampoo is the easy remedy.

● **Sweaty hair**. Whenever hair gets sweaty it lies as it does when excessively oily: when hairs clump together, flippy hair is the rule. Have the hair cut shorter during the warmer months.

● **Harsh water**. If shampoo water has a high mineral content or contains chemicals such as chlorine, your hair may lie poorly. Use rain water or softened water.

The bottom line is: hair that lies poorly is **optional**! Whenever you see it, there is a reason for the problem, and there is a solution. You may have to do a little detective work and spend time educating, but your efforts will be well spent.

C. Permanent Hairloss

The first chapter pointed out that baldness and thinning hair result from a natural process that is largely controlled by genetics and the action of hormones. However, what we do or don't do to our hair also has an impact. Here are the things you can do to minimize hairloss:

● **Shampoo regularly**. Dandruff, dirt, and excess oil combine to make an air-tight cap that chokes off the normal respiration (breathing) that occurs on the scalp. That crusty scalp is a good breeding ground for harmful bacteria and fungus.

● **Massage your scalp frequently**. Blood nourishes the papilla which produce the hair's cells. Anything that promotes an extra supply of blood to the top of the head will be a help. Don't practice the I-will-keep-every-hair-in-place approach:if hair can't be touched, there won't be any scalp stimulation. Avoid whatever hinders the blood flow, such as a tight fitting cap.

● **Watch your diet**. Be sure to have enough protein and important vitamins and minerals.

● **Do not bend the hair at the roots, especially on top**. Don't strain those delicate follicles: pressure on the growth factory is easy to avoid when you let the hair lie the way it wants. Keep the top hair cut on the shorter side: longer, heavier hair bends at or near the follicle. All three haircuts in this book have the top hair cut to a length that allows the hair to lie with the hairgrain.

● **Humor is good medicine**. I've recently read that you can laugh yourself to a state of wellness. I don't know if being in stitches will rejuvenate waning hair follicles, but then, if avoiding stress has an impact on temporary hairloss, maybe there is some help here.

● The best thing scientists have found to stop falling hair? The floor!

● What do they call 10 rabbits in a row, all marching backwards? That's a receding hareline!

Build up an inventory of such jest and you may help someone keep their follicles active—if nothing else, it might keep them from thinking their hairloss is some kind of serious calamity.

D. **Dandruff**

That troublesome white stuff most of us have experienced used to be a very common problem. Today's wash-and-wear haircare has changed this. To explain this impact, you have to know about skin cells.

Every square inch of your skin is continuously shedding old dead cells and forming new replacement cells. On the rest of the body the dead cells don't have anything to prevent their falling away from the skin, but on a head of hair you have 1,000 hairs per square inch to hold those cells close to the skin. Natural oil causes the dead cells to clump together into the little white flakes called dandruff.

Dandruff is just nature's way of telling you you're not keeping your hair and scalp clean enough. This is why wash-and-wear haircare has had such a positive impact—dandruff can't be eliminated, but it can be **controlled** by frequent shampooing. The scalp will continue discarding its worn-out cells; neglect has the cells accumulate into white chunks, but regular shampooing removes them before they're seen.

When dandruff shows up, shampoo twice a day or more until there is no trace of it (have someone inspect your scalp for you). It may take several days to a week before you are on top of it. **Be sure** to use a plastic brush with wide-spaced bristles to give the scalp a good scrubbing before wetting the hair, and use it while you shampoo. When all signs of dandruff are gone, return to shampooing once a day or every other day. If it reappears, resume twice-a-day shampooing with the vigorous scrub beforehand—control is the key word.

Use low pH shampoos for your war on the white stuff: they are effective, yet mild enough to be used twice a day (even ten times a day) without damage to the hair. The different dandruff shampoos on the market are effective, but because of the damage they do to the hairshafts, they are a poor choice. If these dandruff shampoos are used, a low pH rinse or conditioner can help counteract the damage.

Dandruff is more of a problem in the wintertime because of the lack of humidity in the air. Anything that increases the moisture in your environment will be a help.

If the dandruff problem persists and you have worked on it daily,

* * *

If in the past few years you haven't discarded a major opinion or acquired a new one, check your pulse. You may be dead. Gelett Burgess

seborrhea, psoriasis or some other severe condition may be the
problem: go to a doctor or dermatologist and get it taken care of.

E. Split Ends
Hair can get so severely damaged that the ends of the hairshafts split
into two or more "branches". Besides the sick appearance of the
frizzies, this condition is painful. If you took ten strands of barbed
wire and moved them around a little, you would quickly have a tangled
mess that is hard to straighten out—hair with split ends behaves the
same way. When you try to brush out suffering hair the papillae starts
sending pain messages. **OUCH!!!**

To remedy this problem, practice healthy haircare and use low pH
shampoo. Particularly important is a haircut. With this damage, a
haircut is **crucial** because this problem is permanent until the
ends get cut off. This necessary remedy needs patience because of the
growing nature of hair.

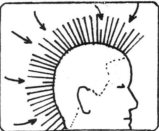

Due to the 3 stages of growth, there are always about 1/4 – 1/3 of the hairs not grown out as long as the remainder: some of these shorter hairs might be split too.

It may take 2 or 3 haircuts (once every couple of months) before all the damaged ends are grown long enough to be cut off.

Cutting off those damaged ends will only be effective if the
haircuttee practices the dos and don'ts. If they continue their
damaging ways, you'll never free them from this condition.

There are many people whose attempts at growing their hair long
always result in frizzy ends. Finer, more damage-prone hair can split
from too much exposure to the sun or to man-made chemicals in the air
and water. The longer the hair is, the longer it has been exposed to
the different sources of split end damage. You have to have strong
hair and careful haircare to grow hair long.

F. Dull Hair
There is a world of difference between hair that gives off a healthy
shine when light hits it, and dull, sheenless hair. Anyone can have
hair that sparkles, but there are dos and don'ts to follow:
- **Mild shampoo.** If you use the strong (high alkaline) shampoos,
expect it to make the cuticle layer curl up. In this damaged condition
any light that hits the hair is diffused; if the armor cells lie flat
as they are supposed to, they reflect light, which is what gives hair
its sparkle. Low pH shampoos make all the difference.
- **Infrequent shampooing.** Natural oils that coat the hair act as a
magnet to any dust or dirt that is around. Keep it clean.
- **Hard water.** Water with a high mineral content can leave a
dulling film on the hair. Use rain water and/or a low pH hair rinse.
- **Inadequate rinsing.** Be sure to get all of the soap suds out;
left in, they dull your lights.
- **Heat and chemicals.** Blow dryers, curling irons, permanents, and
haircoloring all leave the cuticle damaged enough to dull the hair.
Avoid them.

You will get some relief from a mayonnaise or hot oil treatment.
Conditioner or a little dab of lanolin coats the hair and gives it a
little shine. The remedy for this condition is the same as for split
ends: patience + haircuts + proper haircare = healthy, shining hair.

G. **Static Electricity**

Hair standing out from the head when a hat is removed or a comb/brush is used means static electricity has struck again. This problem only shows on straight and wavy hair because this hair normally lies down. Curlier hairtypes are also affected, but this hair always stands out from the head, so the effects are hidden. Here's what can be done:

● **Dryness**. Like dandruff, this problem is worse in the winter when the humidity level is lower. Keep the moisture level up.

● **Natural versus manmade**. Synthetic fabrics such as nylon hats make matters worse than wool or cotton. Handcombing works better than a plastic comb or brush.

● **Lanolin**. A tiny dab of Dusharme helps a lot.

2.8 THE HAIRCUT'S CONTRIBUTION

Healthy hair does not just happen, it's something you get if you take good care. Of all the things that impact on the hair's health, the **kind** of haircut you have is crucial because the right haircut makes the dos and don'ts of healthy haircare **easy** to practice.

A. **Physical Health Benefits**

The two basic ways to give a long haircut demonstrates how the type of haircut you give makes a difference on the hair's health:

1. **The perimeter cut.**

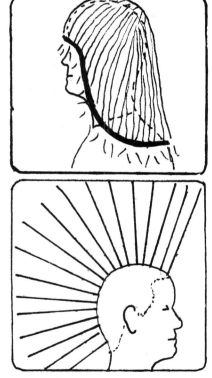

Here the hair is cut only on the edges. You comb or brush all the hair to the back and cut a line across the bottom, or you can cut all around the edges of the hair.

When only the edge hair is cut, a lot of long hair remains.

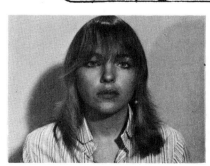

Long hair is heavy hair that wants to hang down.

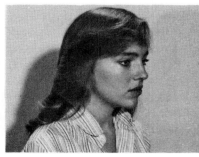

Much time and bending effort is needed to achieve these results.

2. **The long, layered cut.** Here you cut the entire head of hair, leaving about one-half as much hair on the head as the perimeter cut, yet the hair appears just as long:

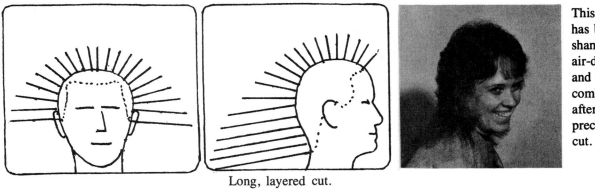

Long, layered cut.

This hair has been shampooed, air-dried, and hand-combed after a precision cut.

Pros and Cons

While it takes more time and skill to give the long, layered cut, it has many healthful advantages over the perimeter cut.

Perimeter Cut   versus   Long, Layered Cut

Use of Kill-o-watts

Perimeter Cut	Long, Layered Cut
A curling iron and/or blow dryer is needed to bend that heavy, hanging hair back. Slow death for the cuticle layers.	With the excess top hair cut off, the hair framing the face lies toward the back naturally, or with just brushing or handcombing. No appliances needed.

Fullness/bending

Perimeter Cut	Long, Layered Cut
The heaviness of long hair causes it to lie flat on top and to bend unnaturally at or near the follicle.	The hair has body and fullness on top, and little or no bending occurs because the hair lies the way **it** wants to.

Shampooability

Perimeter Cut	Long, Layered Cut
Excess hair makes shampooing and drying a time consuming affair. Tangles and snarls makes you want to put it off.	Shampoo and towel dry in a few minutes. Air-dry and you're ready to go. The absence of tangles makes shampooing a breeze.

Follicle Stimulation

Perimeter Cut	Long, Layered Cut
Extra long hair becomes a mess if the scalp is given a massage. Hairspray and a no-touch approach is needed.	Give yourself a scalp massage or handcombing, let the hair be windblown or whatever—the cut keeps the hair in good shape.

Good Riddance

Perimeter Cut	Long, Layered Cut
Some hairs with damaged ends won't be long enough to reach the edge where the cutting occurs: the damage remains leaving the hair tangled and burdensome.	Virtually every hair is cut with this way of cutting. The pain-causing ends are on the floor instead of making life difficult on the head.

B. Mental Health Benefits

Numerous mental health benefits result from the precision haircuts and

* * *

UFF DA!   Norwegian term for burdensome hair.

Make somebody happy today, even if it's yourself.   Anonymous healthy haircare taught here.

● **Carefree hair**. The low maintenance, wash-and-wear haircare these haircuts make possible, result in a concern-free approach to the hair throughout the day: it's much easier to partake of life's little joys when you aren't obsessed with your hair's appearance. People who feel they must keep every hair in place, find these precision cuts meet their no-change needs perfectly; but, they soon see their hair stays in a good shape no matter what happens to it. Yes, the way the hair lies will change throughout the day, but the way it's cut keeps those changes from producing a messy head of hair—the hair is ignorable.

● **A good cut makes you feel better**. A becoming haircut won't lift someone out of the depths of depression, nor does it transform a jerk; but some way or another it does bolster one's mental state. It's hard to pinpoint what it is about a good haircut: for some it is the same feeling you get when you change from grubby clothes; those with sensitive skin like being rid of those bothersome hairs around the ears or neck; for some it feels good to the hands when they move through freshly-cut hair; for some it's being able to look in a mirror again without a frown. Whatever it is, it does make a difference.

● **Less really is better**. A person feels good knowing their haircut maximizes the hair's health while it minimizes the amount of resources, time, and money spent on the hair. With the keep-it-simple approach, you feel better about your corner of the world because you know you're taking good care!

● **A helping hand**. You, the haircutter and teacher of healthy haircare, are using your time in a truly helpful and unselfish way. What do you suppose would be more uplifting: having your hair needs met by someone who cares or by someone whose main concern is money?

● **Spread some quality**. Your haircutting involves you in a skilled work that improves those who receive your best efforts. Whenever a person sees someone at work who knows what to do and how to go about it in the best, most efficient manner, it rubs off and makes you want to do your own work in the best possible way. You won't start out like an old pro, but it doesn't take long when you have a **good** start.

Leo Buscaglia, author of the book Love (Ballantine, 1976), says:
"The purpose of life is to help others, . . . "
The benefits of this type of haircare and haircutting has you dealing with others in a most **helpful** way. The rest of the book covers the haircut how-to, the hands-on way to make hair easy to get along with.

* * *

We are like onions, in layers. Many people live from the outer layer of the onion. They live in what other people think is the thing to do. They are merely imitative or conventional. Their conscience is that still small voice that tells them someone is looking. But we must try to find our True Conscience, our True Self, the very Center, . . . Here lies all originality, talent, honour, truthfulness, courage and cheerfulness. Here only lies the ability to choose the good and the grand, the true and the beautiful.
Brenda Ueland

Falling short of our culture's definition of physical beauty is a genetic gift—you don't have to spend all or some part of your life laboring under the notion that your skin and bone/muscle structure has made you a better person.
Bob Ohnstad

Though we travel the world over to find the beautiful, we must carry it with us or we find it not.
Ralph Waldo Emerson

Nurture yourself.
Message on a button

3.1 THE HAIRCUT CURRICULUM

You will learn to give three basic haircuts. To fill out your bag of skills, you'll be taught several shaping variations for each of these primary ways to cut hair.

A. **The Equal-Length Haircut**.

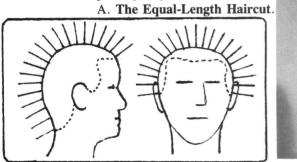 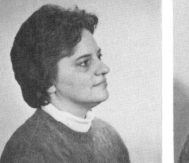 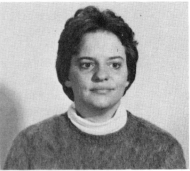

Because this is by far the easiest haircut to give, your learning starts here. The equal-length cut is also the most popular way for men or women, young and old, to wear their hair.

B. **The Long, Layered Haircut**.

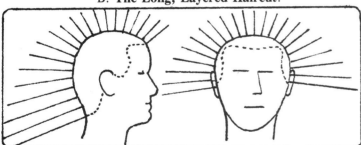 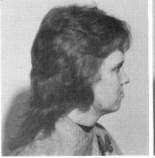 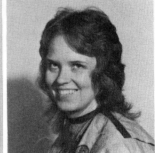

This is the second haircut in your sequence of learning. Hold-off on giving this cut until you have mastered the first one—the longer hair is harder to handle, and this cut has some advanced tool handling.

C. **The Short, Full Haircut**.

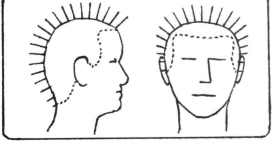 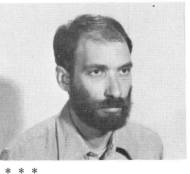 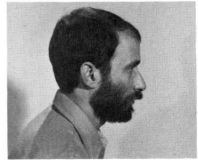

* * *

Give me a fish and I'll eat today. Teach me to fish and I'll eat for the rest of my life.   Anonymous

This longer (more full) version of a short haircut is last, and it is the most difficult of the three. By the time you are comfortable with the first two cuts, you will be in good shape to handle this one.

3.2 YOU NEED A SYSTEM

You may have watched a professional cut hair with a "here a snip, there a snip" approach—they cut all around the head several times without a pattern to their cutting procedure. Good haircuts **sometimes** result from this helter-skelter approach, but it takes a lot of haircutting experience to make it happen.

As a beginning haircutter you need to have a step-by-step, definite system to the way you cut hair. Skim through chapter 8 if you're curious to see the systematic approach that gets every hair cut.

3.3 THE HAIRCUT PROCEDURE—IN A NUTSHELL

Each of the three basic haircuts will have you **pull the hair out** from its normal lying position and **cut off a predetermined amount of hair**. You follow a step-by-step sequence of cuts, moving in a definite pattern over the head of hair. Your hands and tools have to assume some different positions in different parts of the haircut process, and there are minor differences in how you handle the tools with each of the haircuts. Despite the differences, the bottom line is **pull it out and cut it off**.

3.4 HAIR THAT LIES LIKE SHINGLES-ON-A-ROOF

The first day I went to barber school in 1960, my Dad, who has been a barber since the 1920s, gave me these words of haircutting wisdom: Always remember—when you cut hair evenly it will lie like shingles-on-a-roof. His best advice applied to the shorter, clipper-cut styles popular at that time, and it produces the best possible results with the longer, scissor-cut hairstyles common today.

To portray this shingles notion, we'll assume you're giving a haircut to someone with straight or wavy hair. Once a handful of 1,000 hairs (give or take a few hundred) are cut, and the holding hand releases them, the cut hairs bend back into a lying position. The last illustration in this set magnifies the hair's ends so the shingles-on-a-roof idea shows itself.

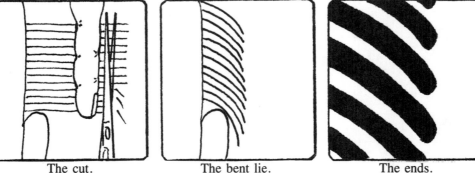

The cut.   The bent lie.   The ends.

The ends of the hair lie like carefully positioned shingles.

The first illustration shows the hair being cut so each hair has the same length—the way it's done with an equal-length haircut.

A long, layered cut has a gradually increasing length around the sides and back. The shingles principle still holds, but the hair ends lie farther from each other than they do with the equal-length cut.

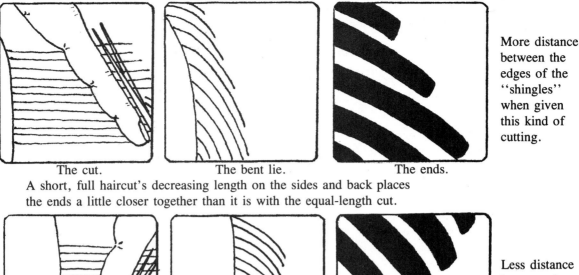

The cut.   The bent lie.   The ends.

More distance between the edges of the "shingles" when given this kind of cutting.

A short, full haircut's decreasing length on the sides and back places the ends a little closer together than it is with the equal-length cut.

The cut.   The bent lie.   The ends.

Less distance between those "shingles" with this way of cutting.

When hair is cut to lie like shingles, those hairs are able to lie in **any direction** and they still have their shingles nature. (The exception to this rule occurs when straight hair is bent against the hairgrain: then the hairs stand out instead of lie down, but at the first opportunity they will return to a more comfortable lie down position.) The fact that those hair ends always blend in with their neighbors is the thing that makes these haircuts so **carefree**—be it windblown, handcombed, or whatever, it still lies like shingles.

Thus far the shingles-on-a-roof comparison has shown single cuts for each of the three basic haircuts. However, a haircut consists of many cuts—if you are not consistent in the length you leave the hair, from one cut to the next, you'll have given a very poor haircut. The goal with any of the haircuts is to have each cut you make blend with the neighboring cuts. This goal is achieved by following the sequence of cuts and pathways each haircut has, and by using the guide-hair aid (explained later). Doing the practice exercises builds the hand skills needed to realize the goal of smooth, precision haircuts.

3.5 THE CUTTING LINE

The main part of a haircut is called bulk-cutting or bulk-removal. The numerous cuts made during this part of the haircut will shorten every hair on the head. As you go through a head of hair making these cuts, one hand holds the hair out from the head while the other does the cutting. The two fingers that hold the hair out are positioned just below an imaginery line, called the **cutting line**. After the held hair is cut, the freshly-cut ends will touch this cutting line while the hair is still in its stand out from the head position.

This cutting line concept is included here so you'll know the overall goal of all the cuts you make during the bulk-cutting part of the haircut. The heavy line in these illustrations is the cutting line you strive for, as the hair is held out from the head for each cut

made during the bulk-cutting. The little marks outside the cutting
line represent the hair that is cut off.

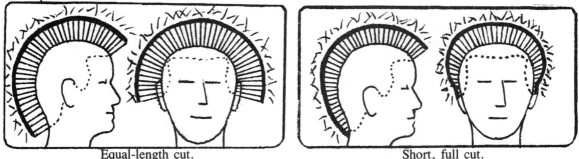

Equal-length cut.   Short, full cut.

These two haircuts have you pulling the hair **straight out** from the
scalp, all over the head of hair while doing the bulk-cutting.

To get the increasing length around
the sides and back of the long,
layered cut, the top hair is cut
with the hair held straight up from
the head. Then the side and back
hair is **pulled up** and cut off,
while you maintain the same cutting
line that was used for the top
hair. Overall, you have this
cutting line.

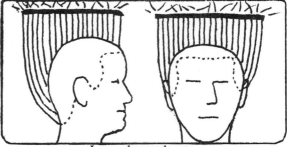

Long, layered cut.

3.6 PREPARATIONS FOR HAIRCUTTING SUCCESS

I'm always on the lookout for ways to make my work a little easier or
more efficient, but some things can't be avoided. That's the way it is
with these preliminaries: they're all necessary to get people-pleasing
results from your first haircut.

● Read through the chapters 1 – 8 as many times as necessary to get a
full understanding of what you want to do and how to go about it.

● Take care in whom you choose for your first haircut. The last
chapter's sections on ''Cutting Childrens Hair'' and ''Haircutter as
Merchant of Change'' are helpful in your choice of the right person.

● Using the information in chapter 7, analyze your haircuttee's hair
and decide the best length and shape for the hair. Reach a
satisfactory agreement on what is to be done.

● Once you know what length is intended for your haircut, do the
practice exercises: they will get you comfortable with the hand-tool
manipulations used during the haircut.

● Heed all the safety considerations that haircutting requires (see
subject index for a review before you begin).

● Set up the best possible working environment. Good lighting and
tools, adequate rest and no distractions makes it much easier.

● Shampoo the hair and dry it. Squeaky-clean hair is a must.

3.7 THE TWELVE STEPS

To cut 100,000 hairs with maximum success, the beginning haircutter
usually needs to go through twelve steps in the haircut procedure.
Some heads of hair won't need all twelve, and with experience, some of

* * *

If you don't know where you're going, you will probably end up
somewhere else.   Dr. Laurence J. Peter

these steps become unnecessary. Assuming you are a beginner and the person you work on needs all of these steps, this is how you'll do it.

Before the Haircut (Steps 1 – 2)

1. Comparing. Give your haircuttee a scalp massage and a handcombing. Show them a mirror—what they see now and what they will see after the haircut is done will prove the value of your new-found skills.

2. Wet the hair. Use a spray bottle to thoroughly wet the hair for your cutting. Expect to re-wet it several times during the haircut.

Cutting Hair (Steps 3 – 10)

Steps 3 and 4 may not be necessary: they depend on how much hair you have to cut off. If you will be cutting off less than 2 – 3 inches, go on to step 5. If your cutting will remove more than 2 – 3 inches, these next two steps will be time well spent.

3. Preliminary edging. Cut an edge-line around the perimeter of the hair. This is done the same as the final edging, but the hair is left a couple of inches longer than what you want for the final length.

4. Approximate bulk-cutting. This step, like the last one, makes your bulk-removal efforts easier. Pull out and cut off the excess hair length in 10 – 12 places all over the head of hair. Again, leave the hair longer than what you want for the final length.

5. Bulk-cutting. This part of the haircut takes the biggest portion of your time and efforts. Despite the time spent here, the cut-by-cut instruction makes this cutting easy to do. With the bulk-removal cuts made here, the main skill to develop is the ability to hold the hair out from the head with the correct holding-hand position. The aids you'll learn make this skill simple to learn.

6. Check for uniform length. Experience eliminates this step, but as a beginner it's an important step. This is done by pulling hairstrands out from the scalp in several locations and measuring their length with a ruler. Major length differences require re-cutting now.

7. Second-time-through. This smooth-off part of the haircut makes the difference between an excellent haircut and a good one. You go over the hair you cut during the bulk-removal, but the holding-hand is held in a different way so you can see and cut any minor length variation. The hair you cut may not fill a thimble, that's usually enough.

8. Final edging. This finishing step has you cutting the edge hairs all around the head. The rule is: cut off very little hair—the hair at the edges has already been cut during the bulk-removal.

9. Extra hairs. Most mature males need their nose, ears, and eyebrow hairs trimmed. Males and females need those stray neck hairs trimmed.

10. Last-minute lookover. You may have to do some last-minute cutting to achieve your best results. With the hair dried and brushed out, give it a good lookover and make any necessary corrections.

After the Haircut (Steps 11 – 12)

11. The after part of the comparison. Brush the hair and let them see how well the "shingles" are lying on the roof. After you give another scalp massage and handcombing, they will know what a positive difference is made with a precision cutting.

12. Instructions for healthy hair. It is not enough to give haircuts that maximize the health of the hair, you also have to spend time and energy teaching the dos and don'ts of healthy haircare. Spend the time to share your knowledge—the results are always positive.

Whether your haircut needs all twelve steps, or some lesser number, you will find this way of going about it gets the job done right!

4.1 HAIRCUT UTENSILS

One of the bench marks of the human race is our ability to make and use tools. For our hair's sake, it's a real good thing: without cutting tools, can you imagine how snarled, tangled and painful most heads of hair would be—**OUCH!!** would be the prevailing expression. The tools you'll learn to use are divided into two broad categories.

A. **Primary Tools**
These tools are all you need to give excellent haircuts.

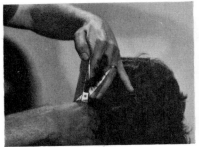

Hands.

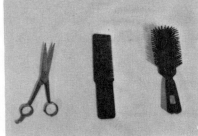

Scissors, comb, brush.

Chair and stool.

B. **Secondary Tools**

These tools, while convenient, are quite optional. You can do a fine job on a haircut without them.

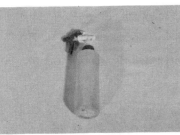

Spray bottle.

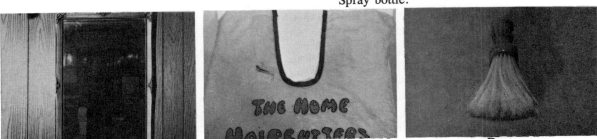

Mirror.   Haircloth and neck clip.   Duster.

4.2 THE CRUCIAL TOOL: YOUR HANDS

Haircutting is above all a **hand** craft. Your use of the tools and the resulting haircuts depend on those mitts of yours. Both hands are crucial, but I think you'll find the left hand is a bit more important than the right in your haircutting efforts. This statement assumes you are right-handed: while 12 – 15 percent of us are left-handed, for purposes of easy description this book had to be written for the right-handers. (Eventually, I hope to write a left-handed version, but until then you lefties will have to flip-flop my how-to directions.)

Assuming right-handedness, the right hand is called the **tool hand** because it does most of the tool handling. Your most important tool, the left hand, is called the **holding-guide-hand—HGH** for short. I will also refer to the HGH as the **holding hand** or **spacer tool**. The first and middle fingers of the HGH are **holding fingers**; the ring and little fingers are called **spacer fingers**.

Holding guide-hand (HGH)   Tool hand.

(1) Holding fingers.
(2) Spacer fingers.

A. **The Work of the HGH**

Your left hand performs three functions during the bulk-removal part of the haircut process.

● **Holds the hair out**. After the right/tool hand combs a tuft of hair up and away from the scalp, your left/HGH hand grabs that hair and holds it out from the head so the tool hand can cut the hair with the scissors.

● **Determines how much hair is cut**. The HGH acts as a spacer tool that regulates how much hair is cut. Your scissors only cut off the hair above the holding fingers of your HGH—the hair beneath the holding fingers is left on the head.

● **Holds the comb**. As the HGH holds the hair to be cut, the right/tool hand transfers the comb to the "V" of the left thumb. With the comb held there, the tool hand can easily handle the scissors as it cuts the hair.

B. **The Work of the Tool Hand**

The right hand performs double duty, handling both comb and scissors. This hand will be kept busy, but not too busy.

● **Combs hair out**. With the hair in a lying position, the right/tool hand combs the hair out from the head so the HGH can grasp it.

● **Manipulate the scissors**. Once the hair is held by the HGH and the comb rests in the "V" of the HGH thumb, the tool hand is free to use the scissors to cut the hair.

When you coordinate the functions of both hands, you will execute one cutting step in the haircut process. This complete step, with all its different parts is called the basic hand-tool manipulation for bulk-cutting. This routine of comb up-hold out-cut off is repeated upwards of 60 times during the bulk-removal (the main part of the haircut) and close to the same number of times during the second-time-through (the smooth-off part of the haircut). The next chapter gives a detailed description of how it's done.

* * *

Knowledge is of two kinds. We know a subject ourselves, or we know where we can find information upon it.
                                                                    Samuel Johnson

4.3 SCISSORS

A. The Parts of the Cutters

(1) Points. (2) Cutting edges.
(3) Thumb blade. (4) Fingers
blade shank. (5) Finger grip.
(6) Little finger brace or
tang. (7) Thumb grip.
(8) Thumb blade shank.
9) Adjusting or pivot srew.
(10) Fingers blade.

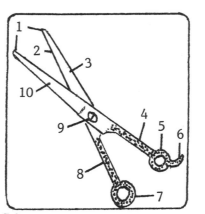

Spend a little time
memorizing these
terms—they are
used quite a bit in
this and upcoming
chapters.

B. Advantages of Haircutting Scissors

The scissors shown above are standard haircutting scissors, called
shears by many professionals. You can use any scissors that cut hair
effectively, but, compared with common household scissors, the
professional version has several important advantages.

● **Using the thumb**

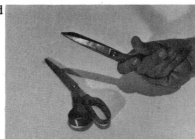

Household
scissors
are
designed
to be
held in
this
position.

When cutting hair, this placement of
the thumb won't allow you to slip your
thumb in and out of the thumb grip in
order to handle both the scissors and
comb with the same hand. The household
scissors' big thumb grip makes handling
the scissors difficult, clumsy, and
possibly dangerous.

The pro model is handled quite different; its design makes this
positioning feel comfortable.

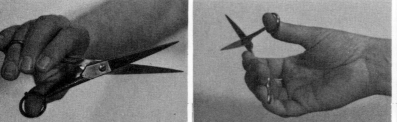

Haircutting scissors in cutting
              position.

Where the scissors rests
when using the comb.

These scissors, handled as shown above, allow the thumb to easily move
in and out of its grip. This positioning makes it easy to move the
scissors in and out of its resting position—where it is placed while
the comb is being used. (More on this in the next chapter.)

● **Points of the blades.**

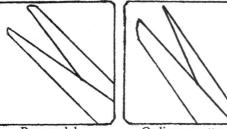

Pro model.   Ordinary cutters.

The pro model has slightly rounded points,
but one or both points on ordinary cutters
are very sharp. This difference becomes
important when the finger-bracing-scissors
method of edge-cutting is used. This
cutting method has the points touch the
skin—with ordinary scissors, that contact
would be more like scratching or stabbing.

● **Saw-tooth cutting edge**
Besides being designed for easy
handling, professional cutters are
also superior because they are made
for cutting hair. Usually one,
sometimes both cutting blades have
a corrugated edge.

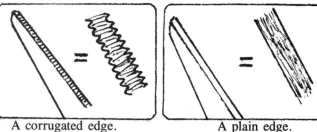

A corrugated edge.   A plain edge.

This rough edge is applied to the blade with a file and it greatly
improves the scissors' cutting ability. Those little teeth grip the
hairs and prevent them from sliding toward the points of the blades as
they are being closed. It is one thing to have scissors do a good job
on paper or cloth, it's quite another to cut 1,000 hairs at one snip.

C. Remedies for Poor Cutting Scissors

You may be using scissors
that, instead of cutting,
pinch the hair between the
closed blades. Or, you may
find the hair slides
toward the points of the
blades.

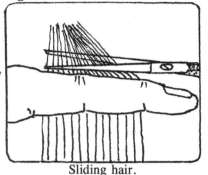

Sliding hair.

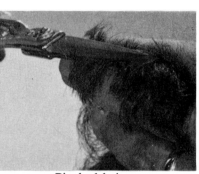

Pinched hair.

Either of these conditions makes your cutting slow and frustrating at
best, perhaps impossible. Here is what you can do about it:
1. **Tighten the adjusting screw**. Because this screw is extra tight,
be sure to use a perfect-fitting screwdriver and back the other end of
the screw against a hard surface such as a vise or a frying pan.

This allows you to put maximum
downward pressure and strength
into tightening the screw—
without the screwdriver slipping
out of the groove. If the pivot
screw gets ruined, you can plan
on buying new cutters.

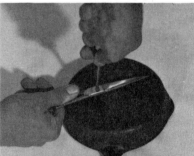

Turn the
screw in a
clockwise
direction.

The right screwdriver will do the job well, but there is a special
tool that makes it easier to keep the screw properly adjusted.

The Lodi Tool is available
at barber and beauty supply
dealers, or by mail-order
from Home Haircutter's
Supply (see the last
chapter).

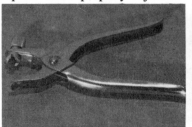

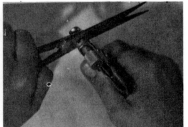

To check for correct adjustment of the pivot screw, hold the scissors
in a horizontal position and open the blades half-way. When the thumb
is removed from its grip, the scissors should open all the way.

* * *

Smart people became that way by asking stupid questions.   Anonymous

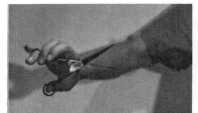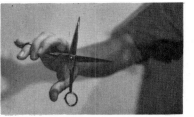

The half-open scissors
open fully.

When you open the scissors a little less than half-way, the blades
remain in that position when the thumb slips from its grip.

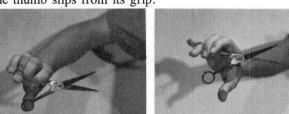

The less-than-half-open
scissors do not move.

This adjustment is needed because the blades of haircutting scissors
have a slight bend that starts at the half-way point of the blades.
This bend gives an extra cutting bite as the blades are being closed.
If the blades are too loose, you can't take advantage of this feature.

2. **The push/pull trick**. As the blades close on a group of hairs,
push a little with your thumb on the thumb grip and pull with your
fingers on the fingers blade shank. This puts extra pressure between
the blades and prevents the pinched hair problem described earlier.

3. **Get your scissors sharpened by someone who specializes in
haircutting scissors.** Beauty or barber supply businesses, usually
found in cities of a quarter-million or more, offer expert sharpening
service. Look them up in the Yellow Pages under barber or beauty
supply and call around (some are open to the public, some aren't).
Home Haircutter's Supply has a mail-in sharpening service, but due to
the cost involved in returning poor quality, unfixible scissors, it's
limited to the scissors they sell (see the last chapter for details).

4. **Spend the money for good quality, professional cutters.** A good
scissors makes the difference between success and frustration. Again,
barber or beauty supply businesses are a source. Home Haircutter's
Supply offers, by mail-order, tools the author knows to be the best
quality at a low to moderate price. Quality cutters are a good
investment—with proper care, they will be passed on to your heirs.

D. How to Keep Scissors Working

When you have good scissors, you'll want to keep them that way.
- Never use them on anything other than hair.
- Never cut dirty hair—be sure it's freshly shampooed.
- Put them in a safe place when not in use.
- Wipe them off after using and give them a few drops of oil between
the blades, including where the blades meet at the pivot screw.

E. Scissors Safety

Keeping the pivot screw at the right adjustment is a crucial safety
consideration. You only move your thumb in and out of the thumb grip
when the scissor blades are closed. Proper adjustment keeps the blades
closed while the thumb is moving in and out—you won't have the thumb
blade accidently flop open as you work around the face. A similar
concern discourages the use of household scissors: the large thumb
grip makes them hard to control as you open and close the blades. A
little slip-up could mean disaster.

4.4 COMB

The comb must eaily lift the hair away from the scalp—some perform
this task better than others.

You have probably seen the traditional
barber's comb. It is a good comb for use
in clipper haircutting, but it doesn't work
well for the haircuts you'll give.

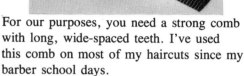

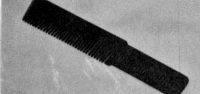

For our purposes, you need a strong comb
with long, wide-spaced teeth. I've used
this comb on most of my haircuts since my
barber school days.

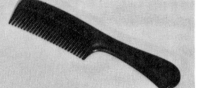

If you are working on extra long hair, on
a thick head of hair, or on damaged hair
that tangles easily, a heavier comb like
this makes the hair easier to handle.

These combs should be available at discount stores, barber and beauty
supply businesses, or by mail-order from Home Haircutter's Supply.

4.5 BRUSH

The boar-bristle brush (with about 2,000 bristles on it) was the
brush to own until plastic brushes (with about 200 bristles) came
along in the 1960s. I try to avoid things made from plastic, but this

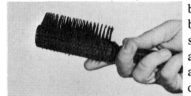

brush has proven to be superior to the old boar-
bristle type. The plastic brush, with its widely-
spaced bristles, works better because it can get
all the way down to the scalp (the old-timer with
all its bristles has difficulty getting past the
outer layer of hair ends).

This tool serves to thoroughly brush the hair before and after
cutting, to massage and to shampoo. You should be able to find one for
less than $3.00 at any drug store.

4.6 CHAIR AND STOOL

The next chapter and the first haircut chapter goes into the specifics
of your position in relation to the haircuttee during the haircut.
This subject is important because you must be able to **see** what you
are doing and **easily** manipulate your hands and tools while
cutting. These objectives are achieved by using a high stool and low
sitting chair for your haircuttee (possibly a cushion too).

On the other hand, if you can buy a used beautician's chair (with a
hydraulic pump in the base), you'll make it easier for your haircuttee
and yourself. Don't buy a barber's chair: they sit higher which works
well for clipper haircutting, but for our haircuts, a lower chair is
needed. Watch the Sunday paper want ads under "Used Business
Equipment". Plan on paying $35 – $75 for one in good operating order.

4.7 OPTIONAL TOOLS

A. **Spray Bottle**
This tool is used with a comb to get the hair soaking wet.

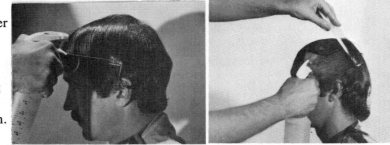

The outer hair is wetted while combing with the hairgrain.

Wet the under hair by combing against or sideways to the grain.

Wet hair is preferable to dry hair because it isn't as likely to slide toward the points as the blades close. And wet hair is neater: when the cut hair falls, it falls away in heavy clumps and doesn't float around, getting on the face and causing the itchies.

In place of a spray bottle, you could use a spray hose connected to a faucet or just wet the hair under the faucet, but, for the money, a spray bottle is a good addition to your tool kit. You will find one at a hardware store or plant shop.

B. Mirror

When you cut hair, you are too close to your efforts to see a sloping neckline, unevenness or heaviness remaining after the bulk-removal cutting.

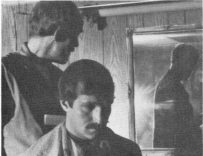

Put a large mirror in your workplace and it increases by 2 – 3 times the distance between your eyes and the hair you're working on.

This little helper is nice to have, however, you get the same effect by backing off 5 – 10 feet and viewing your efforts from there.

C. Hair Cloth and Neck Clip

While not at all mandatory, (a tight collar and whisk broom does the trick,) these two extras are appreciated by most. For youngsters, they prevent a lot of scratching and fidgeting around caused by stray hair, however, some children under the age of 3 or 4 don't want any part of that cloth being around them. These extras can be bought from supply dealers or from Home Haircutter's Supply.

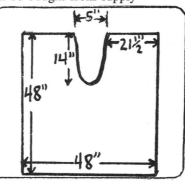

You could also use an old bedsheet cut out as shown and a safety pin. Use a permanent ink pen to inscribe your logo, and include autographs and comments from your haircuttees—your cloth will be as original as every haircut you give.

D. Duster

Getting some cut hair on the nose or neck drives some folks, especially the little ones, half crazy. When they start fidgeting, get rid of the source of their irritation by using an old-time duster (pictured on the first page of this chapter). A shaving brush (from a mug and brush combination) works well—drug stores usually have them, or it might be found at an antique shoppe. Another possibility is a wet wash cloth, or a napkin folded in such a way that the corners stick out from your hand—not real effective, but better than nothing.

5.1 THE "KNACK" FOR USING TOOLS

Many folks believe you must be **born** with some kind of special
ability—called a "knack"—to handle tools with ease. I don't agree.
To me, this is a tired old excuse for staying in the safety of a
narrow rut—for not trying something new.

No, you don't need to have a knack for making things by hand. Yes,
you can get comfortable with hand-tool activities, but, you must:
● Be clearly taught the correct, most efficient way to handle tools.
● Give yourself enough time to gradually improve your skills as you
get more experience—be a little patient during the process.

The first ingredient is my responsibility; the second is yours.
Experience allows you to perfect tool-handling skills. You will go
through a rookie stage where your movements are slow and deliberate,
and you feel uncomfortable and awkward. Be assured: in a short time
handling the tools will be second nature to you—it feels comfortable
and you won't have to think about each little movement of the tools.

5.2 THE BULK-CUTTING PART OF THE HAIRCUT

Bulk-cutting, also called bulk-removal, is the process of cutting the
heavy, hang-down hair that tangles and musses so easily. This part of
the haircut takes the majority of your time as you repeat one tool-
handling procedure about 60 times all over the head of hair (close to
the same number of these hand-tool manipulations are used when you do
the second-time-through cutting). This procedure consists of combing
the hair out from its lying position, grasping the hair with your
holding-guide-hand (HGH), and cutting the hair that protrudes above
your hand. This chapter teaches how to do the bulk-removal for the
equal-length haircut. The slightly different bulk-cutting techniques
for the two advanced haircuts are explained in those haircut chapters.

5.3 POSITIONING THE TOOLS IN YOUR TOOL HAND

Before you can use your tools you have to know how to hold them. (It's
easier to follow these directions if scissors and comb are in hand.)

A. Beginning Position of the Scissors
With the scissors in this position it's easily tucked away so the tool
hand can also handle the comb.

● Place your ring finger in the finger grip, between the first and second joints. Bend the finger at both joints. (The "first joint" is the first one from the finger's tip.)
● Place your slightly bent little finger on the tang, close to the first joint.
● The middle finger bends at the second joint, and the first joint—where the shank rests.
● The first finger is extended forward, both joints slightly bent—the shank rests at the first joint.

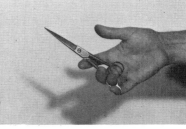

B. Move the Scissors to its Resting Place

● Pull your middle finger in toward the palm of the hand, sliding the scissors to the "V" of your thumb: the resting place.
● Your first finger goes along and helps direct the cutters to the "V".
● Keep your ring finger stationary—it acts as a pivot point for the scissors' trip.
● The tang slides out till it's positioned between the little finger's tip and first joint.
● Extend your thumb forward and clamp down on the scissors, holding it firmly.
● The first and middle fingers can relax.

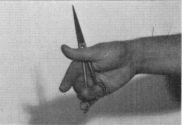

C. Grasping the Comb

● Extend your thumb and first finger.
● Grasp the comb.

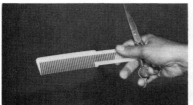 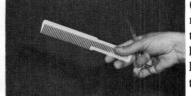

(Use your middle finger too if the hair is long, heavy, or thick.)

5.4 THE BASIC HAND-TOOL MANIPULATION

Work slowly at first. With practice the nine small steps of this basic manipulation will flow together and seem like one quick movement. To explain all the steps that go into one bulk-removal cut, we'll examine the first cut in an equal-length haircut. Wet the hair and comb it forward on top.

STEP 1

Insert comb about one inch into the hair, with the teeth lightly scraping the scalp. Hold the comb flat on the scalp.

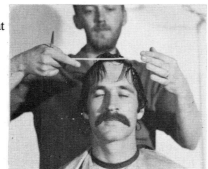

From your viewpoint it looks like this:

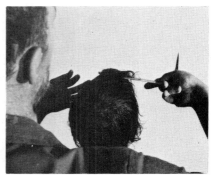

I hear and I forget. I see and I remember. I do and I understand.

Chinese Proverb

STEP 2
Lift the comb
and hair
straight up
from the scalp.
Leave some hair
protruding above
the comb. Hold
the comb in that
position.

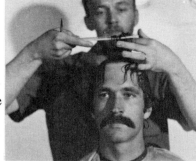

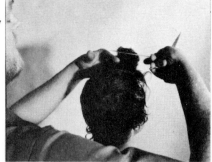

The way
you see
it.

STEP 3 As the last photos show, while you lift up the hair, your
HGH gets ready to grasp the hair.

When the hair is
combed up, grasp
the hair between
your holding
fingers, below
the comb.

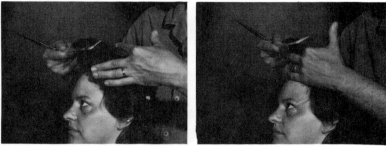

Exactly where you grasp the hair depends on the length you intend to
leave the hair. Chapter 7 tells how to make this decision, and section
9 in this chapter has practice exercises that enables you to repeat
the same length producing position each time the hair is grasped.

Once the hair is in hand, the holding
fingers apply a pinching pressure and
a slight upward tug on the hairs to
keep them standing straight out from
the scalp.

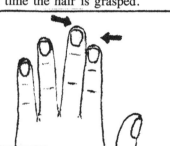

The first and
middle fingers
are held in
this position.

If the holding
fingers are
on top of each
other, the
hair is not
held straight
out as it
should be.

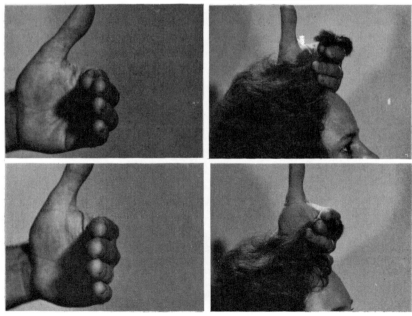

STEP 4 Lift the comb up through the hair above your holding

fingers. Then transfer the comb to the ''V'' of your HGH thumb, and
hold it with the thumb.

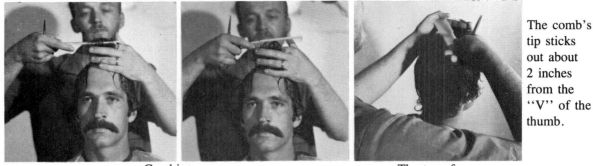

The comb's
tip sticks
out about
2 inches
from the
''V'' of the
thumb.

Combing.   The transfer.

With practice you'll have enough speed to grasp the hair as the comb
makes a non-stop journey up through the hair, to the ''V' of the thumb.

STEP 5 Move the scissors from its resting position to the cutting
position.

● Pull in your little finger
(it's on the tang) as you. . . .
● Hold your ring finger (in
the finger grip) stationary.
● The blades slide out and
stop at the first joint of
the middle and first fingers.

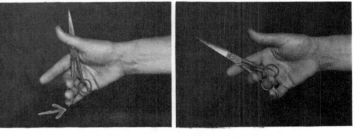

● Insert
thumb in
its grip
and open
blades.

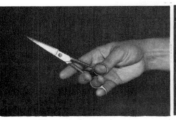

Insert thumb.   The cutting position.

The ring finger is bent at the second joint and is positioned in the
grip at the first joint, which is also bent. The first two fingers are
also bent, with the shank positioned at their first joint. The thumb
is placed in its grip between the tip and the first joint: any farther
and it's hard to slip the thumb out again—if it isn't in far enough,
you won't have good control as the blades are being opened or closed.

STEP 6 Position the blades on both sides of the held hair.

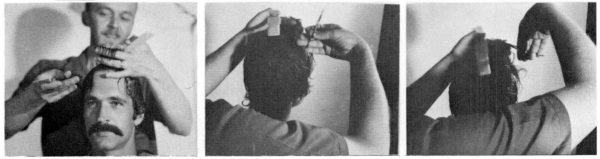

With practice you will combine this step with step 5. While
positioning the scissors in your tool hand, you position your arm and
wrist so the blades are on both sides of the held hair.

Always start cutting at the finger tips and proceed toward the big knuckle of the holding fingers. For support, rest the bottom-side of the thumb blade on the top of the middle finger that is holding the hair. You can do your cutting without this resting guide, but you increase your chances of snipping your holding fingers.

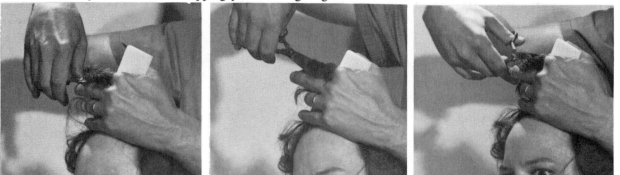

Position the blades flat on top of the holding fingers.

Do not position the blades these ways.

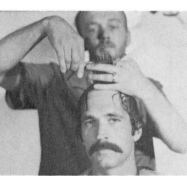

STEP 7 Cut slowly and carefully. It may take a couple of snips to get from the finger tips to the "V" of the holding fingers. You have better control if you make more than one cut.

Maintain your HGH position with the pinching pressure (between the holding fingers) after you have cut the hair.

STEP 8 Return the scissors to its resting place. With the scissors closed, remove your thumb from the thumb grip. The middle finger (which is still bent around the shank at the first joint) pulls the scissors into the resting position at the "V" of the thumb. The ring finger is a stationary pivot point during the trip. The tang should be positioned between the little finger's tip and the first joint when the scissors is at rest. As you reach for the comb, extend the thumb (which holds the scissors in place) and first finger to grab the comb.

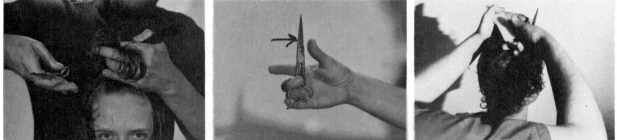

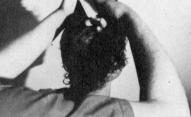

Thumb out.   To the resting place.   Reach for comb.

Throughout this step, maintain the position of the HGH with the pinch pressure applied.

STEP 9 Your tool hand takes the comb from its resting place in the HGH. Pivot the bottom of your HGH out and away from you while you maintain the pinching pressure. Position the comb flat (teeth lightly scraping the scalp) at the base of the held hair. Move the comb toward you about an inch: at the same time, release the hair between your holding fingers. You are ready to comb up another tuft of hair and to go on to your second basic manipulation.

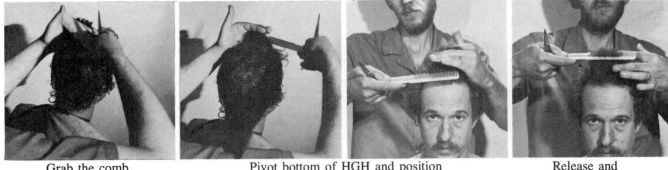

Grab the comb.   Pivot bottom of HGH and position   Release and
                                comb.   comb up.

Holding the hair until you are ready for the next comb up and cut,
eliminates snagging the comb in the hair and it insures that you stay
on the same pathway, cut after cut. In time you will gain enough speed
to lift your HGH up and release your grip on the hair, while you slip
the comb into position for the next comb up. Until then, the pivot
movement gets the job done as you are building speed.

5.5 THE COMB-AWAY METHOD: THE OTHER WAY TO DO IT

This variation of the basic manipulation is necessary to learn because
the comb **always** has to move through the hair, going either against
or sideways to the hairgrain. When the comb moves through the hair in
the same direction as the grain, all you do is comb the hair **down**:
the HGH can't grasp the hair if it's combed down.

All bulk-cutting can be done with the standard method, but when it
comes to the second-time-through part of the haircut, the comb-away
method is well used. In addition, you may want to employ this approach
for the sake of variety, or it may feel more comfortable on some parts
of the bulk-removal.

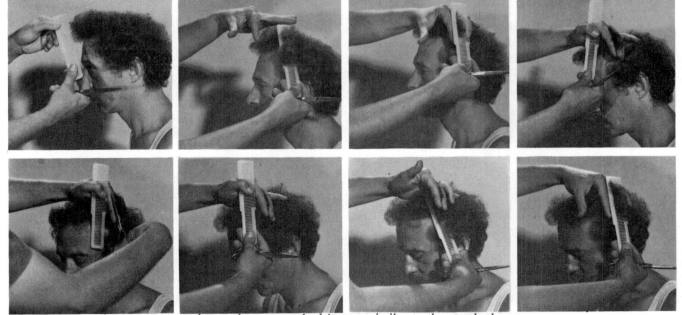

As you can see, the comb-away method is very similar to the standard
method. The minor differences are:
● The teeth of the comb point, and the tool hand moves away from
you.
● When the comb is in its resting place, the teeth point away from the
"V" of the thumb.

● When you insert the comb at the base of the hair held by the HGH, you can see exactly where the comb is placed. Also, you don't need to pivot your HGH up to get the comb to the base of the held hair.

This way to use the tools requires extra care because the points of the scissors move toward the head or face, especially when the cutters are in their resting place and you are manipulating the comb: go slow and be aware of the points of the scissors as they move about. (I've never had any problem, but I am always mindful of where those points are while the comb is being used—you do the same.)

5.6 THREE AIDS TO EQUAL-LENGTH CUTTING

Now that you know how to manipulate hands and tools for one cut in the bulk-removal process, you are ready to learn how to do all the haircut's basic manipulations so the job gets done **right**. Leading off, we have the **primary aid** toward the goal of a consistent length to the hair.

Aid 1 With every cut made in the bulk-removal process, the bottom of your HGH rests on the scalp.

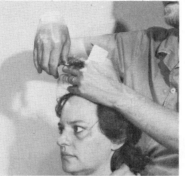
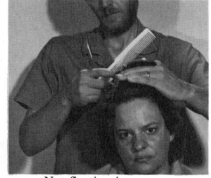

Something to lean on.   Not floating in space.

Different cutting lengths require different HGH positions:

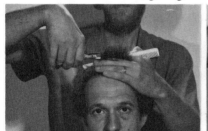
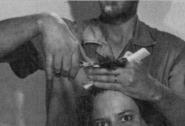
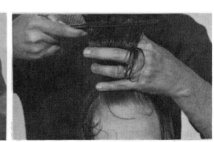

1 inch cut.   2 inch cut.   3 inch cut.

The shorter the hair is cut, the closer the fingers of the HGH are spaced and the more palm touches the head. On the shortest version, the inside of the spacer fingers are also touching the scalp. The longer the hair is left, the farther apart the fingers on the HGH are spaced and the palm doesn't touch the head—just the bottom edge of the hand and little finger is in contact.

The important thing to keep in mind when giving an equal-length haircut is: choose a length for the hair, find the HGH position that produces that length when you cut, then **repeat the same holding hand position throughout the entire bulk-removal process**. (Chapter 8 shows where and how the hair's length can be altered, but this rule is the key to equal-length haircutting.) The practice exercises at the end of this chapter enable you to repeat the same length-producing HGH position, time after time just on the basis of **how it feels**.

Aid 2 You will follow a systematic sequence of cuts in the pathways and sections of the head. With this system you can't miss a hair on the head. Skim through chapter 8 to see how you go about it.

<u>Aid 3</u> An advantage of cutting hair in pathways is that you usually work beside a pathway that has already been cut—this cut hair is the hair you use as a **guide**. You comb up and hold a little of the already-cut hair—the guide-hair—along with the uncut hair.

For example, say all the cuts are completed in the first pathway.

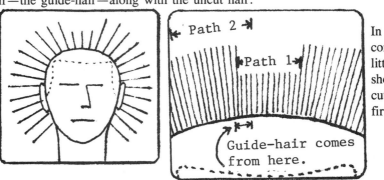

In Path two, the comb picks up a little of the shorter, already-cut hair from the first path.

The scissors point to the already-cut guide-hair from the first pathway. The longer hair that protrudes above the holding fingers is the uncut hair from the second pathway.

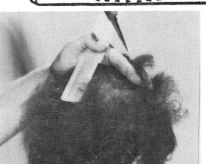

Because of the sequence of paths you cut on the top section, the guide-hair shows at the "V" of the holding fingers on some paths, and at the finger tips on other paths. As you work on the sides and back, guide-hair always appears at the "V".

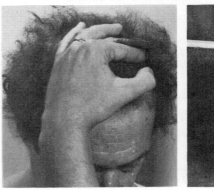

Guide-hair at the "V".   At finger tips.

When your HGH is in the correct length-producing position, you should have about 1/8 – 1/4 inch of guide-hair protruding above the holding fingers—cut the longer, uncut hair to match the shorter, already-cut guide-hair. But **don't** cut any of the guide-hair.

There are two main advantages to using the guide-hair aid:
● It keeps you on the right path, making it impossible for you to drift around the head.
● It shows you how much to cut off on the basis of how much was cut off on the last pathway. However, remember the most important way to achieve a consistent length with each cut, is for you to have the bottom of your HGH in contact with the scalp—this allows you to manipulate your HGH on the basis of how it **feels**.

* * *

Next time you feel like complaining, remember your garbage can eats better than 30 percent of the world's population.   Anonymous
A man is rich in proportion to the things he can afford to let alone.
                                                Henry David Thoreau

Live simply that others may simply live.   Quaker proverb

5.7 MISCELLANEOUS HAND AND TOOL INFORMATION

A. The Holding-Guide-Hand

1. Holding the hair out from the head. When giving an equal-length haircut, you pull the hair **straight out** from the head.

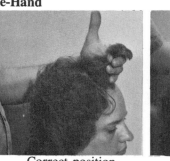
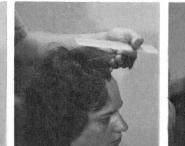
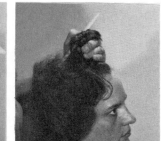

Correct position.　　　　Incorrect positions.

2. Pulling tension. Be sure that all the hairs between your holding fingers are held with a slight pull-up tension that keeps all the hair straight.

Maintain a continuous, gentle pressure so no hairs buckle.

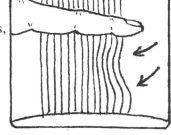

Those buckled hairs would have a longer length than those hairs held straight.

3. Working on curly and kinky hair. With straight or wavy hair the amount of pull-out pressure you put on the held hair can vary from a little to a lot and it won't make any difference. However, curly and kinky hair are like coiled springs and must be **consistently** stretched out for cutting.

It is important that you maintain (as much as possible) the same pulling tension on the hair, snip after snip. Without a consistent pull-out pressure, the hair is cut to uneven lengths.

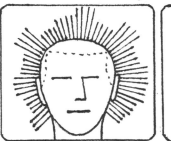
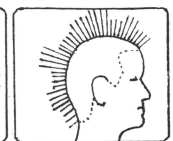

This unevenness can be removed during the second-time-through part of the haircut, but at that time you should be making minor adjustments.

4. The HGH conforms to the shape of the head. When you leave the hair longer, the bottom of the HGH and little finger rest on the scalp; when the hair is left 2 inches or less, more of the palm of the hand and the inside of the little finger (and ring finger too on short-short lengths) rest on the scalp. These lean-on-the-head positions result in the bottom of the HGH conforming to the shape of the head: the holding fingers **effortlessly** conform too.

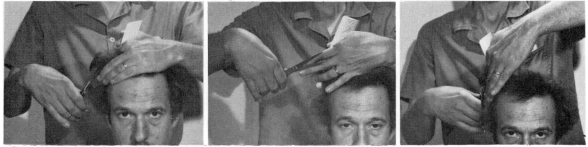

Correct position is relaxed.　　　　Incorrect positions require extra effort.

The way the HGH conforms to the head depends on the shape of the head in the area you are working on. Heads come in all shapes, but you will find most heads have four fairly flat areas, and five curved areas on the haircutting part of the head. These are the four flatter areas.

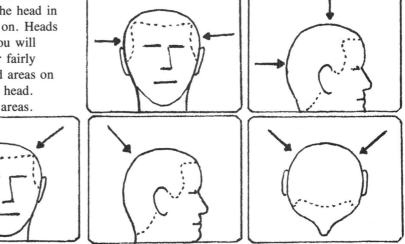

The five curved areas.

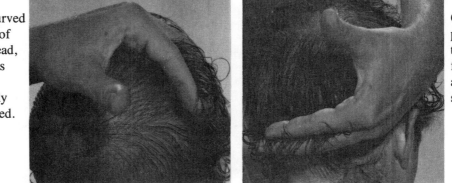

The flat areas won't give your HGH any problems—the holding fingers easily conform to the underlying shape of the head. The curved areas can be a little difficult for some beginners—these rounded areas need a slightly different HGH position than what is used on flat surfaces.

On curved parts of the head, fingers are slightly rounded.

On flat parts of the head, fingers are held straighter.

If you have difficulty getting your HGH to conform to the curved areas of the head, all you do is cut an extra pathway between the two already-cut pathways on the curved area. For example:

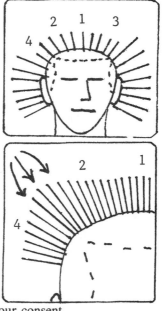

You are cutting the top of the head—an area of both flat and curved surfaces. You cut pathways 1, 2, and 3 with ease. With pathway 4 you encounter a curved surface and your HGH doesn't conform as it should.

After cutting pathway 4, you may find the hair is left longer than it should be. To get these hairs all the same length, cut an extra pathway between paths 2 and 4. This extra path overlaps both of the two already-cut paths.

* * *

Remember, no one can make you feel inferior without your consent.
Eleanor Roosevelt
My life is in the hands of any fool who makes me lose my temper. Anon.

Pathways 2 and 4 serve as guide-hair for the hair that needs to be cut. The guide-hair shows at the "V" and tips of the fingers—cut the longer hairs in the middle. (A glance through the photos for the top pathways in chapter 8, section 4-A will illustrate this further.)

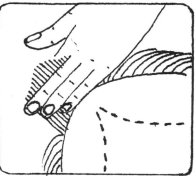

Most beginners are able to get their HGH to conform to the curved areas; if you have problems, just make an extra path between the two already-cut paths.

5. The impact of the head shape.

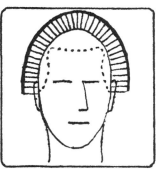

Because the HGH conforms to the shape of the head, the head's shape will determine the overall cutting shape— the cutting line you give to the hair. There is a wide variety of head shapes and each shape produces a different cutting line on an equal-length haircut.

To determine head shape, spend a minute before the haircut familiarizing yourself with that noggin. In various places on the head of hair, firmly push down on the scalp with both hands: the shape of your hands tells you the shape of the head hidden by the hair.

A skull may have minor bumps such as the knowledge bump located at the back of the head where the spine meets the skull. Ignore these small irregularities.

B. The Comb and Easy Hair Handling

1. **Untangling the hair**. Be sure the hair is free of tangles and snarls by thoroughly brushing and combing before cutting. The comb must be able to move through the hair without obstructions: to achieve this you may have to give damaged hair an approximate haircut (see section 8). This procedure removes most of the damaged ends that slow you down, and it makes things less painful for your haircuttee.

2. **Combing out the hair**. When you work on straight, wavy, or somewhat curly hair, comb the entire head of hair before you begin cutting. Comb out and away from the cowlick: on top, you comb toward the front; on the sides and back, you comb downward.

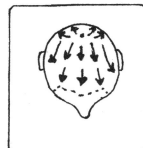
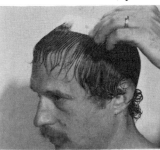
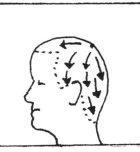
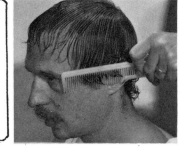

After you finish all the cuts in a pathway, you **always** recomb the hair as shown above—before you start your next pathway.

Combing the hair this way has the hair lying with the hairgrain for the most part. When you make the cuts in the pathways, the sequence of cuts goes in an opposite direction: this approach makes it easy to comb the hair out from the head so your HGH can grasp it.

3. **What to do when the comb gets snagged**. When the comb travels through the hair either against or sideways to the hairgrain, it may snag in the hair from time to time. The practice of maintaining the pinching pressure between your holding fingers until the comb is reinserted into the held hair eliminates most snag problems during the pathway cutting; but beginning a new pathway presents some problems. These aids get you going without snags.

● **The helping-hand method**. Use this approach when you start cutting a pathway or whenever your comb snags. When the comb runs onto some uncooperative hair, place your HGH in front of the snag (or below it if you have a snag around the sides or back).

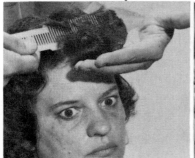 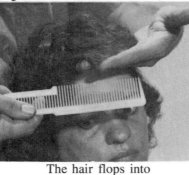 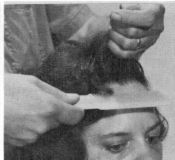

The HGH lifts up the hair so the comb can be placed at the base of the held hair.

Lift the comb out and toward the HGH.

The hair flops into the palm of the HGH.

The comb is reinserted.

A variation of this method is to grab the edge-lying hair with the HGH, lift it up, and insert the comb at the base of the held hair. If the comb lifts out without snags, you can proceed. If it snags, flop the hair back into the HGH as shown above, and you're on your way.

● **The sideways trick**. With this technique you can start out anywhere on a head of hair. It's particularly useful when you start the pathways above the ears—the tops of the ears are easy to catch with the comb if you do it any other way. Place the comb so that the teeth touch the scalp.

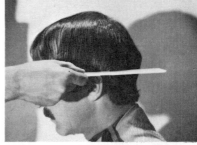

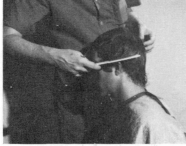 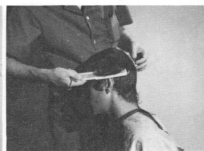 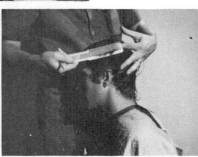

Gently scrape the teeth against the scalp as you move the comb a couple of inches to the left or right.

Lie the comb flat (parellel to the head) and insert it about an inch into the hair.

Lift the comb away from the head. The HGH grasps the hair before the comb is out of the hair.

This procedure works well; however, there may be times when the comb gets snagged as you start the lift-out: use the helping-hand method.

C. Scissors Handling

1. **The thumb grip is too big.**
While I've never heard of
someone's thumb being too large
for a thumb grip, there are
many thumbs too small for the
grip. Reducing the size of the
thumb grip is easily done with
a rubber reducer placed into
the thumb grip's opening.

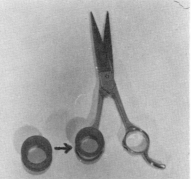

Barber or
beauty supply
dealers have
this handy
aid. Home
Haircutter's
Supply sends
one with each
scissors sold.

2. **Cutting curly and kinky hair.** Straight and slightly wavy hair
stand straight out from your holding fingers, making it easy to
position the scissors' blades on both sides of the held hair. Curlier
hair is less cooperative because it wraps around the tops of your
holding fingers. The remedy is simple enough, but somewhat
time-consuming. All you do is gently (very gently) scrape the tops of
your holding fingers with the points of the blades as you slide the
scissors into its cutting position—this insures that **all** of the
held hair gets between both cutting edges.

Cutting
curly
hair
requires
this
slower
scissors
handling.

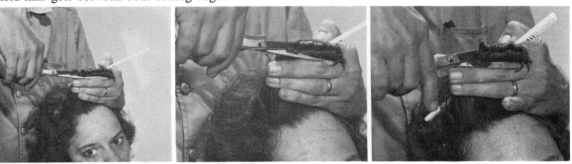

3. **Positioning the wrist and arm.** To wield the scissors
effectively and comfortably, the wrist must be bent while you hold
your arm out and away from the body.

Cutting the hair on top
is a little arm-tiring,
but you need the line of
vision shown here.
Cutting around the sides
and back has the more
relaxed position shown
in the photo at right.

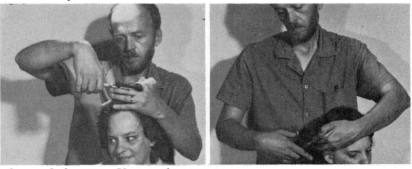

4. **Positioning yourself and your haircuttee.** You need to see
clearly what you're doing and to handle your tools with ease. The
recievers of your efforts need to be comfortable. A beautician's chair
meets both of these needs, or you can use a high stool, a chair, and a
cushion too if needed. The haircuttee sits on the stool for cutting on
top, and on the lower sitting chair for the sides and back. You stand
straight or with knees slightly bent, using whatever position you need
to maximize your vision and ease with the tools. These positions make
your tool handling as relaxed and comfortable as possible:

* * *

Rules for living: have your yesterdays filed away; your present in
order; and your tomorrows subject to instant revision.   Anonymous
Ulcers come from mountain climbing over mole hills.   Anonymous

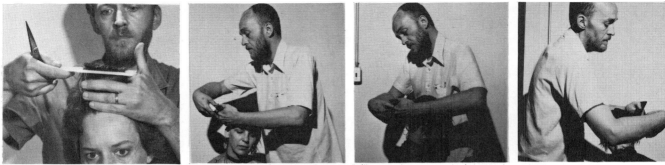

Stool for the top.   A lower sitting chair for the sides and back.

Extra help comes from the haircuttee moving their head to positions convient for you—it may be a little tiring on the neck to hold their head to one side or the other for a period of time, but your ease in handling the tools is the most important consideration.

5.8 THE OPTIONAL STEP: THE APPROXIMATE HAIRCUT

If you must cut off a lot (2 – 3 inches or more) of hair, you need to make the hair easier to handle before you do the bulk-cutting. This can be accomplished by using the familiar basic tool manipulation to cut the hair at 10 – 15 evenly spaced locations around the head. There is a quicker method, shown here.

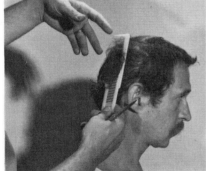 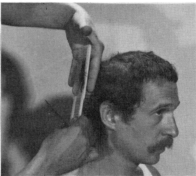 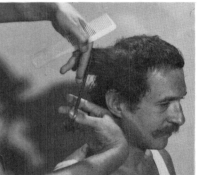

Insert comb   Grab the hair   Comb to resting place;
and lift out.   below the comb.   position scissors and cut.

The last photo shows the hair being cut above the holding fingers; it could also be cut on the inside part of the fingers. Be sure to leave the hair at least 1 inch longer than what you want for the final cutting length on the bulk-removal part of the haircut. If the hair needs approximate cutting, you might want to give it a preliminary edge-cutting too (the next chapter has the how-to).

5.9 PRACTICE MAKES PERFECT

Let's say you decide to learn to drive an automobile. How do you go about joining the ranks of the car drivers? You would probably enroll in a driver's education course and get as much practice as you can. This book is your "driver's education" and here you learn how to practice the skills you've read about.

While cutting hair you'll position and move your hands/arms in a variety of ways quite unfamilar to you. This means you'll start slowly and feel awkward (just like it was when you learned how to drive). The following exercises minimize the awkwardness, and help build muscles, coordination, and speed. Spend at least an hour a day for one week

getting comfortable with the skills in these exercises—**it will be
time well spent**.

The first two exercises train you to hold your HGH in whatever
length-producing position you may want—with practice, the **feel** of
your hand tells you it's positioned correctly. Use one or both of
these first two exercises; each has its own advantages.

Exercise 1 **The Practice Board**

Get two pieces of plywood or any kind of scrap wood about 1 foot
square. Drill a 1/4 inch hole in the center of each. Take two pieces
of cord or heavy string about 6 inches long and tie a knot in one end
of each. Feed the strings through the holes in the boards.

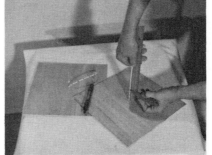

Using a ruler, mark off 1/2 inch
intervals on the strings with two
felt-tip pens. Alternate the
colors; i.e., every half inch
is marked in blue, and every
inch is done with a red pen.

Use clay or putty to build up a curved surface on one of the boards.

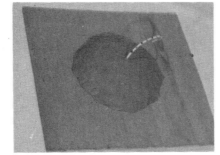

Have you figured it out yet?
The board with the clay on it
simulates the curved areas of a head;
the board without the clay represents
the flatter areas of a head.

You use your tool hand to hold the string out, while the HGH grabs the
string over and over again—until you are 100 percent familiar with
how the hand feels at different length-producing positions.

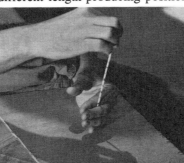
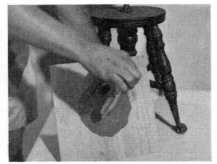

Lying flat it's similar
to the top of the head.
In a vertical position
it's like the sides
and back of the head.

Practice at all the 1/2 inch marks between 1 – 3 1/2 inches.

The advantage of this exercise is that you don't have to take up
someone's time as you do with the second and third exercises—you can
just sit and fiddle with your strings whenever you like.

The next two practice exercises bring more realism into your
preparation efforts. Try to do these exercises on the person who will
receive your first haircut. Because longer hair is clumsy and hard to
handle, the patient person on whom you practice should not have hair
longer than 4 – 4 1/2 inches.

Exercise 2 **Comb and Ruler**

Here you practice the basic hand-tool manipulation, and a little of the comb-away method as you follow the sequence of cuts for the bulk-removal on the equal-length cut (see chapter 8). However, instead of handling the scissors you'll have a ruler on a nearby table. As you follow the sequence of cuts, paths and sections, each time you comb up the hair and position your HGH in the length-producing manner you want, you reach for the ruler and measure your results.

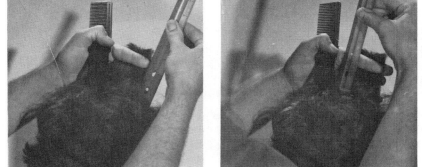

Be sure to measure to the **top** of the first finger in these two places.

Once or twice through all the cuts should enable you to consistently manipulate your HGH into the length-producing position you want.

Exercise 3 **The Dry Run**

With this exercise you polish up your HGH skills, but more important, you get some practice with hands, scissors, and comb working together.

Go to Chapter 8 and follow the step-by-step photos of the bulk-removal and second-time-through cutting. Go through every step as if you were giving a haircut, but close the scissors in **front** of the hair held by the HGH. Do this once a day for several days before your first haircut, and you're in excellent shape for your initial effort.

Also practice the helping-hand and sideways comb handling methods—use as needed as you go through the bulk-removal process.

5.10 THE SLOW WAY TO HANDLE TOOLS

The hand and tool manipulation information in this chapter will have you snipping along in the best, most efficient way possible. If you have trouble getting your hands and tools to work together as described, there is a simpler, but much more time-consuming way to do it. Keep in mind, **every beginner** has some difficulty developing the muscles and coordination necessary for using their hands in this new way. Don't be easily discouraged.

The objective for your first haircutting experience is good results, not to be super efficient with your tool-handling. This slower way will accomplish your objective.

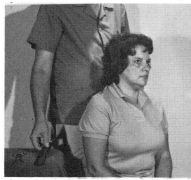

The scissors and comb are on the table— reach for the comb.

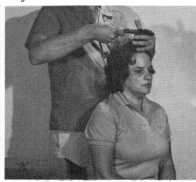

Comb up the hair and position the HGH.

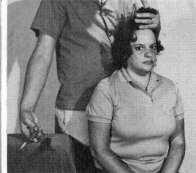

Place comb on table and pick up scissors— maintain HGH position.

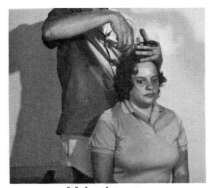

Make the cut.

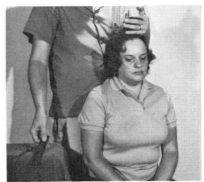

Place scissors on
table. Pick up comb
while you maintain
the HGH position.

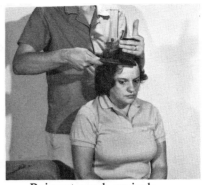

Reinsert comb an inch
further into the pathway
and you're ready for the
next comb up and cut.

As you can see, more than a little patience is needed—this approach
doubles or triples your cutting time. Do yourself and your haircuttee
a favor by becoming adept at the faster method as soon as possible.
Millions have learned how to handle tools this way—you can too.

* * *

Christianity: Therefore all things whatsoever ye would that men should
do to you, do ye even so to them: for this is the law of the prophets.

Matthew, 7:12

Judaism: What is hateful to you, do not to your fellowmen. That is the
entire law; all the rest is commentary.   Talmud, Shabbat, 31a

Buddhism: Hurt not others in ways that you yourself would find
hurtful.   Udana-Varga, 5, 18

Confucianism: Surely it is the maxim of loving-kindness: Do not unto
others that you would not have them do unto you.   Analects, 15, 23

Taoism: Regard your neighbor's gain as your own gain and your
neighbor's loss as your own loss.   T'ai Shang Kan Ying P'ien

Zoroastrianism: That nature alone is good which refrains from doing
unto another whatsoever is not good for itself.   Dadistan-i-dinik 94, 5

Islam: No one of you is a believer until he desires for his brother
that which he desires for himself.   Sunnah

Brahmanism: This is the sum of all true righteousness: deal with
others as thou wouldst thyself be dealt by. Do nothing to thy neighbor
which thou wouldst not have him do to thee hereafter.   The Mahabharata

Love thy neighbor as thyself.   The Great Commandment

If these (the Golden Rule and Great Commandment) were followed out,
then everything would instruct and arrange itself; then no law books
nor courts nor judicial actions would be required; all things would
quietly and simply be set to rights, for everyone's heart and
conscience would guide him.   Martin Luther

The test of our progress is not whether we add more to the abundance
of those who have much; it is whether we provide enough for those who
have too little.   Franklin D. Roosevelt

There are some men who, in a fifty-fifty proposition, insist on
getting the hyphen too.   Dr. Laurence J. Peter

The whiteman knows how to make everything . . . but he does not
know how to distribute it.   Sitting Bull

By virtue of being born to humanity, every human being has a right to
the development and fulfillment of their potentialities as a human
being.   Ashley Montagu

All that we send into the lives of others comes back into our own.

Edwin Markham

6.1 EDGE-CUTTING USES A DIFFERENT APPROACH

Edge-cutting (also called edging) is quite different from bulk-cutting. Here you comb the hair down and cut a little hair close to the skin.

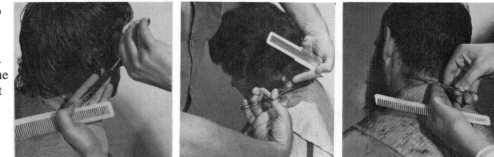

With the bulk-removal done before you do the edging, the hair around the edges are already shortened. Because of this, a minimum cut-off is all that's needed to get the edge hairs in good shape.

6.2 MAIN RULE FOR EDGE-CUTTING

While there are some differences in the edge-cutting you do on the two more advanced haircuts, the main rule for cutting edge hair on an equal-length haircut gives you a good introduction to the way the hands and tools are used on all three haircuts. When doing the edging on the equal-length cut, you comb the hair down and out, straight away from the hairline, and you make your cutting line **conform** to the shape of that hairline. In other words, your cuts are parallel to the underlying hairline. To do this, you must be aware of the shape of the hairline that lies beneath and above the edge hair you're working on.

You must comb the hair back, up and away from the hairline to be able to see it: always take the time to see what you have to deal with.

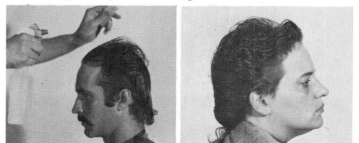

This is a typical hairline:

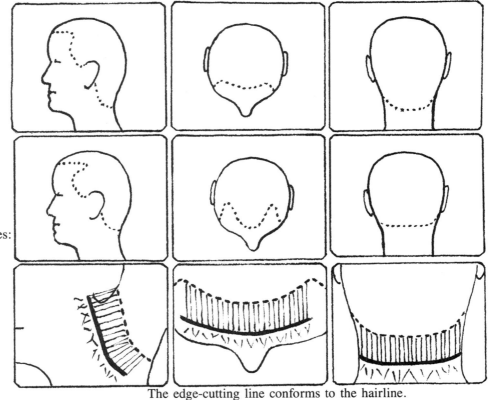

However, there are wide variations from the typical; this is one of the many less common hairlines:

Here the heavy line represents the edge-cutting line; the dashed line represents the underlying hairline:

The edge-cutting line conforms to the hairline.

There are a few minor exceptions to the main rule for edging:

● **Hair covering the ear**.
If your cutting conforms to the shape of the hairline in this area, you'll have the edgeline shown on the first illustration. Some like it this way, however, most prefer the edgeline shown on the right.

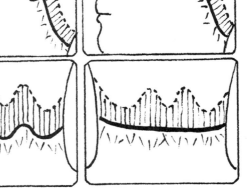

● **Neck edgeline**.
Besides the common straight across neckline shown above, many have a wavy shape (with a ducktail and a Type 2 hairgrain). The edgeline can be cut to conform to the shape but most prefer a straight line.

● **Bangs**. Bangs are normally cut to conform to the shape of the hairline.
Looking down on the top front of the head, these illustrations show the cutting line following the hairline:

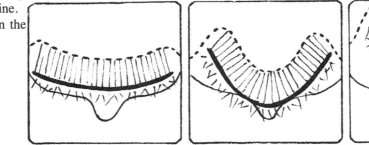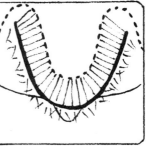

When you work on someone with hair that grows straight forward onto the forehead (about 10 – 20 percent of the time) the edging can be done as shown above or you can use a couple of other approaches.

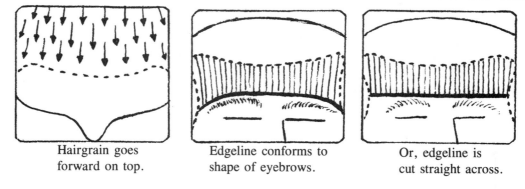

Hairgrain goes forward on top.   Edgeline conforms to shape of eyebrows.   Or, edgeline is cut straight across.

6.3 THE TWO TIMES TO CUT HAIR AROUND THE EDGES

Usually you cut the edge hair once, sometimes twice, during a haircut.
1. **Preliminary cutting**. This edging is done if you have a lot
(three inches or more) of hair to cut off. This cutting makes the
bulk-removal easier—that excess hair is hard to handle, and a minute
or two spent cutting it around the edges beforehand is time well
spent. The same cutting methods are used for this edging as for the
final edging. The difference here is that you leave the hair at least
an inch longer than what you want for the finished length on the
edges—a little margin for error that is taken care of during the
bulk-cutting and when you do the final edge-cutting.
2. **Final edging**. This edge-cutting is almost always done after you
have finished the bulk-removal and the second-time-through (smooth it
off) cutting. The next section explains why it isn't **mandatory** to
do this part of the haircut, and the last chapter's section on cutting
children's hair tells when you should avoid this procedure; but, I
think you'll find the finished product is always improved when you
trim those edge hairs a little.

6.4 HOW MUCH HAIR TO CUT OFF?

With preliminary edging you may have to cut off quite a bit of hair;
most of your final edging will have you cut off as little hair as
possible. This minimum cutting means just snipping off the edge hairs
that are a little longer than the majority of edge hairs. If you need
to cut more, usually less than 1/8 inch is quite sufficient. To
explain why this minimum cutting approach is used, you have to know
what happens with equal-length bulk-cutting.

Assume that your bulk-removal left
the hair 2 inches long: comb hair
into the edge-cutting position and
the tips of those hairs that grow
at the hairline now lie 2 inches
inches from the hairline.

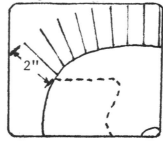
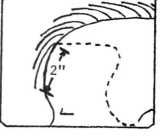

The same holds true anywhere on the
head of hair—the hair ends lie
2 inches from the hairline where
ever the hair is combed straight
away from the head of hair.

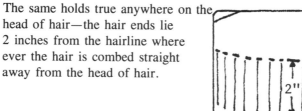
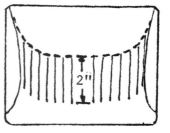

With a smooth bulk-cutting, the tips of the edge hairs are parallel to the hairline they are combed away from: they're already in the basic shape you strive for when you follow the main rule for edge-cutting. (This is why you can skip the edging if you give a haircut to a child who can't sit still.)

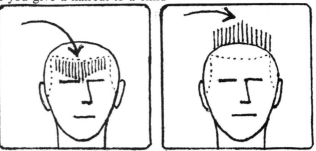

If you didn't cut the hair evenly during the bulk-removal, when the hair is combed down for edging there will be some extra long hairs. Go back through that area and redo the bulk-cutting: you'll find the long hairs are gone when you comb the hair down a second time.

Because the bulk-removal is smoothed off by the second-time-through cutting, **before** you begin the edging part of the haircut, there is little chance you'll find the edge hairs as uneven as shown above. Nevertheless, if you should see a bunch of edge hairs longer than their neighbors, check to be sure the bulk-cutting in that area was done right.

Assuming the edgeline is free of bulk-removal boo-boos, you cut off the small number of hairs that will always be a bit longer than the majority of hairs on the edges—a little smoothing off does it.

The heavy, solid lines represent edge-cutting lines:

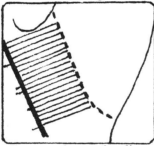
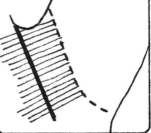
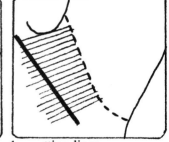

Correct edge-cutting line.   Incorrect edge-cutting lines.

Going back to the example of the 2 inch equal-length haircut, if you were to cut off an inch of edge hair, you would undo your bulk-cutting efforts. Cutting edge hair 1 inch shorter creates the unevenness shown in the far illustration.

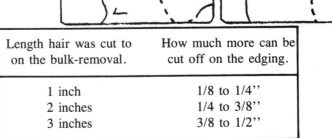

If you feel the need to cut the edgeline a little shorter than just trimming off the longer hairs, stay within these guidelines.

Length hair was cut to on the bulk-removal.	How much more can be cut off on the edging.
1 inch	1/8 to 1/4''
2 inches	1/4 to 3/8''
3 inches	3/8 to 1/2''

There are three exceptions to the above guidelines—these areas offer some flexibility:

1. **Neckline hair**. If you have given a 3 inch haircut to a person with a short neck, and the three inches of hair below the neck's hairline does not fit the person well, or if they prefer not to have the neck hair brushing against their collar, as much as 2 inches of

the neck hair can be cut off. If you do cut the neckline hair an inch (or more) shorter, you should taper those bottom hairs to avoid a bowl-cut appearance to the hair (see the chapter 8, section 5, for the 2-step tapering procedure).

2. **Hair in front of and covering the ear**. Here you may need to cut off 1/2 inch (or more) of the perimeter hair in order to have the straight across edgeline that was shown on page 73 of this chapter. If you cut off an inch of this ear-area edge hair, you will probably need to do a little 2-step tapering to have the hair lie well.

3. **Lower temple-area hair**. If you give a longer version of the equal-length cut, the lower temple region hair may have to be cut shorter than the minimum approach. This hair can flop forward into the corners of the eyes if left too long.

6.5 BULK-CUTTING LENGTH AND ITS EFFECT ON THE LENGTH OF BANGS AND EAR-AREA HAIR

For the guidelines below to hold true, assume that the hair being cut is straight and fine-textured with a Type 1 hairgrain. Understand that these lengths are only approximates: factors such as a receding or low hairline, big or small ears, all have an influence on these averages. After you have done the bulk-cutting that leaves these lengths, you can expect the hair to lie accordingly.

Bulk-removal length	Hair covering ears	Bangs
3 inches	To the bottom of the ears or slightly longer.	To about the eyebrows or a little longer.
2 inches	About 1/2 – 2/3 of the ear covered.	About 1/2 – 2/3 of the forehead covered.
1 inch	Top 1/5 – 1/4 of ear covered.	Hair lies 1/5 – 1/4 down the forehead.

As the next section indicates, these approximate lengths don't hold true when you are working on some kinds of hair other than straight, fine, Type 1 hair.

6.6 THE EDGELINE YOU CUT WILL SHRINK

The edgeline you cut while the hair is wet will raise up and seem to shrink when the hair is dry. While wet hair can stretch a little and then resume its normal length when dry, the effects of hair's elasticity are hardly noticeable. Of more importance are:

A. The Springy Nature of Wavy, Curly, Kinky Hair
You pull these types of hair down to their cutting position; when they are cut and resume their normal (out and away from the scalp) way of being, the edgeline rises quite a bit—the curlier the hair, the more it rises up from the cutting position. For example, you give a curly head of hair a 3 inch cut. When you do the edging on the bangs, the hair is pulled down to eyebrow level. After cutting, the hair is released and it rises up to its normal, out from the scalp position.

* * *

Curiousity cures ignorance.
                                                                    Anonymous
Anyone who stops learning is old, whether at twenty or eighty. Anyone who keeps learning stays young.
                                                                    Henry Ford

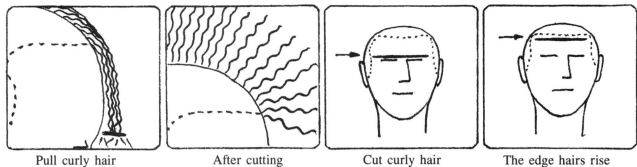

| Pull curly hair to cutting line. | After cutting it springs back. | Cut curly hair at this point. | The edge hairs rise to here or higher. |

B. The Direction the Hair Wants to Lie

With curly and kinky hair, hairgrain does not have much, if any, impact on the lying direction of the hair. With straight or slightly wavy hair, hairgrain has a major impact on the direction the hair lies. How the hairgrain causes the edgeline to shrink is illustrated by the two examples below.

● If the hair has a Type 2 hairgrain, it greatly affects where the hair ends up lying as it covers the ear.

For example, say you give a 3 inch equal-length cut, during the edging you pull the hair straight down over the ear and cut the edge hairs a little below the ear.

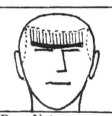

When that hair lies naturally toward the back, the edgeline rises about halfway up the ear.

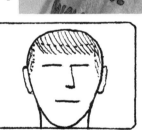

● If the hairgrain on the top of the head goes off to one side and you cut the edgeline at eyebrow level, expect the hair to lie about halfway on the forehead.

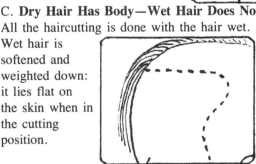

C. Dry Hair Has Body—Wet Hair Does Not

All the haircutting is done with the hair wet.

Wet hair is softened and weighted down: it lies flat on the skin when in the cutting position.

When wet hair dries, the added weight is gone: the hair then has body and the edgeline rises.

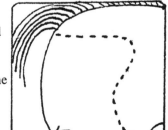

How much this factor causes the hair to shrink up depends largely on the texture of the hair. Fine hair tends to be limp whether it is wet or dry, so there won't be much effect on this hairtype. Coarse hair is a different story: if your edging was done to 3 inch long coarse hair, you could expect the hair to shrink up as much as 1 inch.

As you can see, where the hair finally lies around the edges is determined by several different factors. With this information you can make an educated guess on the subject, but cutting the edge hair so it lies **exactly** where it's wanted requires you to "feel" your way:

● Do not cut off too much edge hair at one time. You can always cut

off more hair, but once it is too short, . . . You are always better off
to be extra cautious with how much you take off the edge hair.

● Plan on modifying the bulk-removal length on the second and third
haircuts you give a person. The length the hair is left on this
cutting determines the length of those edge hairs. First haircuts
are always something of a learning experience: with the second effort
you will zero-in on the best cutting length.

6.7 FOUR EDGING METHODS: HOW TO DO THEM

The bulk-removal involved only two basic hand-tool methods. Edge-
cutting, while it takes only 10 – 15 percent of your haircutting time,
requires you to learn four different methods. Don't despair. There are
good reasons for this, and because you already have learned the how-to
for bulk-cutting, you will find these techniques quite easy to learn.

A. The Modified-Bulk-Removal Method

As the name implies, this edge-cutting is done with the same basic
hand-tool manipulation used for bulk-cutting. There are a couple of
minor differences:

(1) With bulk-cutting, you always combed the hair straight up and out
from the scalp. With this edging method you comb the hair more forward
(about 45 degrees) and grasp the hair between your holding fingers.

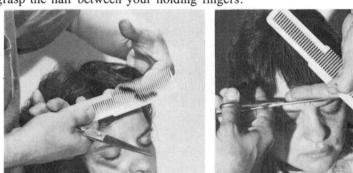

Comb the hair forward.
Then pull the hair down
and straight away from
the hairline. Cut off
the hairs longer than
the majority.

(2) When bulk-cutting, you cut paths through the hair. With this kind
of cutting, you will comb only the hair that is a **little behind the
hairline** forward, down and away from the hairline, then cut off a
small amount of the hair. You move around the head, repeating this
procedure on the neighboring edge hair.

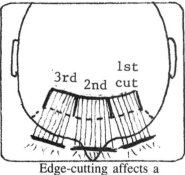

Edge-cutting affects a
small part of the hair.

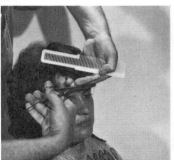

Begin at the front,
left of the bangs.

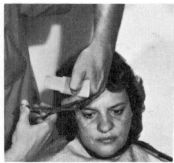

And move around the
head.

(3) To hold the hair down and away from the hairline, the HGH is
used in a slightly different manner than what you're used to. There
are three ways to handle your spacer tool; which one you use depends
on the length the hair was left during the bulk-removal:

● Medium lengths. If the hair is 2 – 2 1/2 inches long, tuck your spacer fingers in under the hair you are holding. The little finger rests against the hairline and helps insure that your holding fingers also conform to the shape of the hairline.

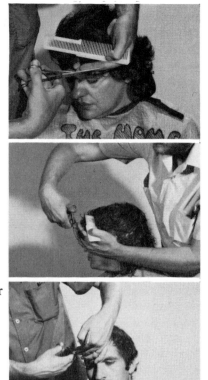

● Longer hair. With hair longer than 2 1/2 inches, you need to slide your holding fingers out on the hairshafts until you reach the desired cutting position. You won't have anything to lean on, so you must be extra aware of the shape of the underlying hairline, and make your holding fingers conform to it.

● Shorter hair. When you're dealing with hair shorter than 2 inches, you won't be able to tuck your spacer fingers under the held hair—there isn't enough room. Position the holding fingers so they reflect the shape of the hairline. Let the inside of the spacer fingers rest on the skin.

This less than 2 inch, more than 2 inch rule is flexible in that it depends on the size of your fingers. Small fingers could go as short as 1 1/2 – 1 3/4 inches with the tuck under approach; big fingers might need more than 2 1/2 inches of length in order to fit the spacer fingers under the held hair.

While this method of edging can be used on most parts of your edge-cutting, I find it particularly useful for edging around the face and especially the bangs. It leaves the edge hair with a softer appearance than do the next three methods.

B. The Finger-Bracing-the-Scissors Method

This method works well when the hair is on the short side. It can be used on any of the edging except for the hair that covers the ear—the last method is best for that edging. This method is often used to trim the neckline and bangs on the equal-length cut, and it will always be used for trimming men's sideburns. There are two ways to do it:

1. **The standard way**. The tool hand has the same beginning position for comb and scissors as used for bulk-cutting. Comb the hair down—straight away from the hairline—so the hair lies on the skin. Put the comb in its resting place, and position the scissors in your tool hand for cutting. With the blades open, use the first finger or two of your HGH to support and steady the scissors as you **gently** scrape the skin with the dull outside part of the thumb blade's point. As you position the scissors' blades on both sides of the hair to be cut, the point of the thumb blade slips under the hair to be cut, while the finger blade remains visible.

* * *

How long is a minute? It depends on which side of the bathroom door you're on.   Anonymous
Some people see stumbling blocks; others see stepping stones.   Anon.

Once the thumb blade's point touches the skin, slide the scissors forward to get the hairs to be cut between the blades. Steady the scissors with your HGH during this procedure.

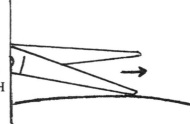

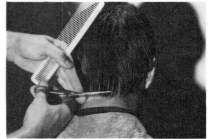

Make the cut, then place the scissors back in its resting position. Grab the comb again, and you are ready for the next comb down and cut.

2. **The upside-down way**. This approach is the same as the standard way, except that here you see the back of your hand, while the standard approach has the inside of your hand visible.

This method allows you to cut in the opposite direction than you did with the standard way. Note the different position for the finger that does the bracing.

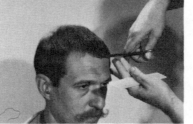

Upside-down.   Standard.

Here are some more how-tos:

● When cutting hold the blades perpendicular to the skin, as the above photos show. The **back** of the blade is in contact with the skin.

Never cut with only the point of the blade touching the skin.

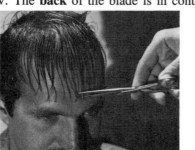

Never cut with the side of the blade in contact with the skin.

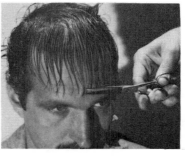

● You cut at a right angle to the hair's combed out, lying position.

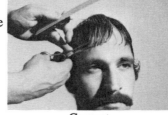

Correct.

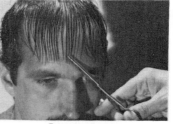

Incorrect.

● Do your cutting with short, 1/2 – 1 inch snips rather than one long snip. Make a cut, open the blades, move the cutters forward another 1/2 – 1 inch, make another cut, etc. Re-comb whenever the hair gets bent away from its straight out from the hairline lying position.

* * *

A study of police records show that a woman has never shot her husband while he was doing the dishes.   Anonymous

If you can smile when everything is going wrong, you're either a nitwit or a repairman.   Anonymous

Too many people are willing to carry the stool, when the piano needs to be moved.   Anonymous

● As much as possible, you should cut against the hairgrain. For example, if the grain goes this way on top:

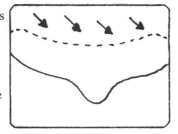

Make the cuts go in this direction:

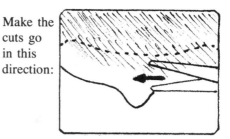

C. Scissors-And-Comb Method

This edging technique is useful with shorter hair, especially where the hair's grain is strong enough to prevent the hair from lying straight away from the hairline for the edge-cutting you want to do. The comb, **handled by the HGH**, bends the hair away from its natural lying inclinations as the tool hand manipulates the scissors. Here's how it is done:

● Comb through the hair toward the edgeline for an inch or two. Stop the comb when the ends of the comb's teeth are where you want the edgeline to be—some hairs will protrude from the ends of the teeth.

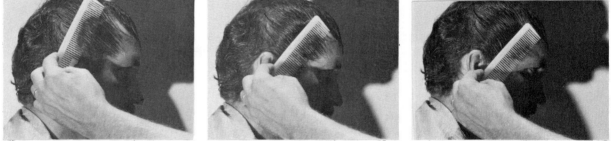

The comb-through.   The hold.

● With the comb in this holding position, lift the teeth of the comb about 1/4 inch away from the skin while you keep the backbar of the comb pressed against the hair and scalp. This pivoting movement with the comb pulls the hair that protrude beyond the comb's teeth away from the skin. Now you have ample room to position the scissors' blades on both sides of the hair to be cut.

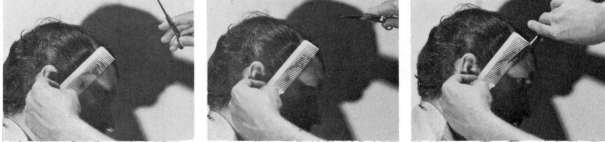

The lift-out.   The cut.

This lift-out procedure usually gets all of the hair to be cut, away from the skin for your cutting ease. However, some hairs may slip from the comb—cut the remaining hairs held by the comb, then repeat the comb through and lift-out to get **all** of those ends cut.

* * *

Love doesn't make the world go round. Love is what makes the ride worthwhile.
                                          Franklin P. Jones
Love is a fruit in season at all times, and within the reach of every hand.
                                          Mother Teresa
The only abnormality is the incapacity to love.
                                          Anais Nin
Take away love and our earth is tomb.
                                          Robert Browning

Repeating this procedure a second time requires the use of guide-hair. You need to look close to see the already-cut hair. The shorter guide-hairs are seen against a background of longer hair.

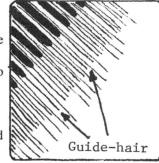

Stop the comb when the teeth are at the guide-hair. Pivot the comb out, then cut.

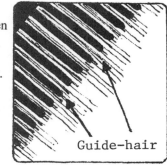

D. Pull-And-Cut Method

With this way of edging, your HGH resumes its role of holding the hair (with a new twist to it,) and your tool hand manipulates both the scissors and comb again. This method works well if your bulk-cutting left the hair 1 1/2 inches long or more. The pull-and-cut can be used on any part of the edge-cutting, but there are three occasions when I find it to be the **best** way to go: preliminary edging; the edging on the hair that comes down over the ear; and edging longer hair that doesn't want to lie straight away from the hairline. This is how you go about it:

● Hold the comb and scissors in the tool hand. The teeth of the comb lightly scrape the scalp as you comb through the hair at a right angle to the hairline.

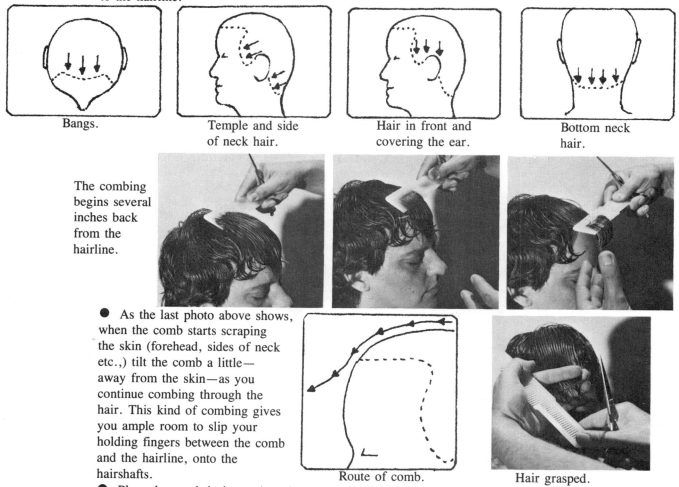

Bangs.

Temple and side of neck hair.

Hair in front and covering the ear.

Bottom neck hair.

The combing begins several inches back from the hairline.

● As the last photo above shows, when the comb starts scraping the skin (forehead, sides of neck etc.,) tilt the comb a little—away from the skin—as you continue combing through the hair. This kind of combing gives you ample room to slip your holding fingers between the comb and the hairline, onto the hairshafts.

Route of comb.

Hair grasped.

● Place the comb in its resting place and apply the pinching pressure between the holding fingers as you slide the fingers out to the length-producing position you want. Position scissors for cutting and snip away on the **inside** of the holding hand (cutting the hair this way is new twist referred to earlier).

These photos show the pull-and-cut used on the side of the neck. Each cut was preceded by the comb-through described on the previous page.

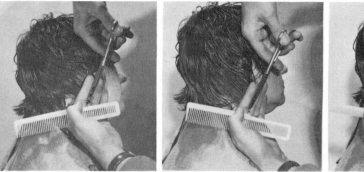 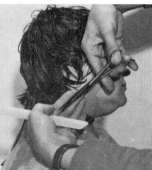

● The middle finger and spacer fingers touch the skin: you want to cut as close to the hair's lying position as possible.

● Make the cuts on the inside of the hand whenever you use the pull-and-cut. You will notice in the haircut chapters I occasionally do the cutting **above** my holding fingers: this is just a little different approach I use (without thinking) when working on longer hair. Don't try to follow my old habits—do your cutting on the inside of the fingers. (For sake of consistency, I would have re-shot those few photos to show the cutting done the right way, but it wasn't possible to get those folks used as models back to the photographer's studio.)

6.8 SEQUENCE OF CUTTING

Like bulk-cutting, edge-cutting needs a systematic approach to have every edge hair cut to the right length. Glance through the edging part of the equal-length haircut chapter; the cutting moves from a cut area to a neighboring uncut area (with minor exceptions) in a specific sequence of cuts all around the the head. Here again, you use the guide-hair aid; but remember, you have to be aware of the shape of the hairline and have your holding fingers and cutting conform to it.

● The preferred pull-and-cut method has the guide-hair show up at the fingertips or at the "V" of the holding fingers, depending on what part of the edging you are working on.

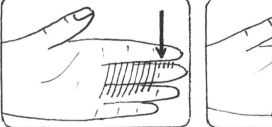

When I do the cutting above my holding fingers, my fingers slide out far enough on the hairshafts so the shorter hairs (from the last cut) fall from my holding finger's grasp. Then I stop the slide-out and cut the hairs above the fingers.

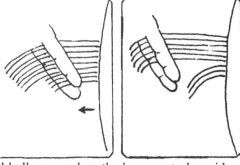 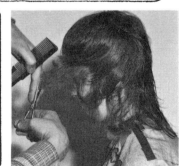

● When using the modified-bulk-removal method, one cut alongside of another, the guide-hair shows as it did for ordinary bulk-cutting.

● As you comb through the hair when using the scissors-and-comb method, overlap your combing so some shorter guide-hair from the last scissors-and-comb cutting is included. Stop the comb-through when the guide-hair is at the tips of the teeth. Pivot the comb and cut the longer hair—your cutting will be a continuation of the previous cut.

● The finger-bracing method uses guide-hair to the extent that each time you make a short snip and move forward for another, your cutting will be a continuation of the line made by the last cut.

6.9 WAYS TO PRACTICE EDGING

When you're ready to practice the edge-cutting methods you should have already gone through the practice exercises for bulk-removal tool handling. This additional practice wont take much time: spend 5 – 10 minutes a day for a few days to go through the same "dry run" practice used for bulk-cutting. Practice all four edging methods, and you'll be well prepared. If you feel the need for a little more realism and you have a willing recipient, these relatively easy kinds of cutting help perfect your skills.

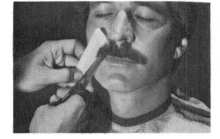

A. Finger-Bracing-the-Scissors

Do a little mustache trimming. Comb the hairs down and cut them off so the bottom is even with the top of the lip.

B. Scissors-and-Comb

If the mustache comes down around the corners of the mouth, you can also do some practice with this edging method. All longer mustaches, except the handlebar variety, are trimmed this way.

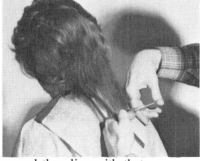

Comb all the hair that grows alongside the corners of the mouth toward the corner. Hairs that stick out from the comb are trimmed off. The pink of the lip at the corner is the point at which the hair is cut.

C. Modified-Bulk-Removal

Somebody always needs their bangs trimmed a little. The last chapter has additional how-to information on bangs trimming.

D. Pull-and-Cut

Find someone with long hair who would like a little trimmed off the bottom back hair. Shampoo the hair and thoroughly brush it toward the back.

Have the person tilt their head forward and cut from one side, straight across to the other side. Let the hair air-dry, then brush it again. Now with the head in an upright position, trim off any stray long hairs.

* * *

I think somehow, we learn who we really are and then live with that decision.

Eleanor Roosevelt

When you have practiced these cutting methods you'll have all the major tool skills needed to get excellent results on your first equal-length haircut.

Edge-cutting, like bulk-removal, can be accomplished by using the easier, but slower approach that has a nearby table to lie the tools on when they are not in use. This one-tool-at-a-time approach can be used with any of the edging methods except for the scissors-and-comb method. Remember, being efficient with your tool handling is not crucial to your success. The main objective is to get the hair evenly cut. The slow or the fast way gets you to the objective, but you make it much easier on yourself and your haircuttee if you take the time to develop these more efficient methods.

Before you learn to determine the right length for hair, the finishing touches and a couple of minor skills need to be covered.

6.10 DRYING THE HAIR

Before you get into the last steps of the haircut, the hair has to be dried. You will be looking over the hair and checking for any less than smoothly-cut areas: heavy, wet hair does not allow you to **see** imperfections. There are a couple of ways to get the hair dried.

A. The Slow Dry
If the hair is to be air-dried, first give the hair a thorough towel-drying. Then comb or brush the hair so it lies with or is slightly bent away from the hairgrain. This comb out is necessary because as the hair air-dries, the hair will "set": if it is lying in different directions before the air-dry, it will do the same after it dries. This slow drying causes a head of wavy hair to become more wavy, even curly, because wet hair clings together—this multiplies the hair's tendency to be wavy or curly. If the haircuttee prefers less wavy or curly hair, use the next drying method.

B. The Fast Dry
If your haircuttee is in a hurry or they want straighter lying hair, thoroughly towel-dry the hair, then. . . .

Drum-dry the hair with the fingers:

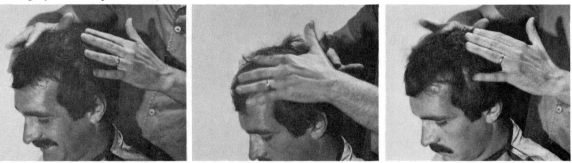

A rapid drumming dries a head of hair in less than five minutes—when it would have taken as long as an hour to air-dry. Also, it feels good to the scalp and it's a good workout for the arms. Handcomb the hair into its preferred lying position after it's dry, or nearly so.

This kind of drying adds extra body or fullness to the hair. If the hair is just air-dried, it is weighted down from the moisture and it sets close to the scalp. When you drum the hair dry, it fluffs and dries farther from the scalp.

If the hair is flippy after you have the hair lying the way it wants to, now would be the time to take care of it.

6.11 HOW TO DEAL WITH FLIPPY HAIR

When I see someone walk in the shop with flippy, misshapen hair, most
of the time it is caused by poor, uneven cutting. Other causes include
excess length that makes the hair bend from its preferred lie, and
things like oiliness and damaged hair. The precision haircuts you
learn here rule out the biggest cause for flips, but then, it takes
only a few seconds to check a flippy area to be sure your bulk-cutting
has left the hair evenly cut. Use both the first-time-through bulk-
removal and the second-time-through HGH positioning. If you find it
uneven, trim as needed.

  After you are sure the flippy area is cut right, try a little hair
bending. You need a brush with widely-spaced teeth and a spray bottle
with warm water in it. Wet the hair and brush through the flip area.

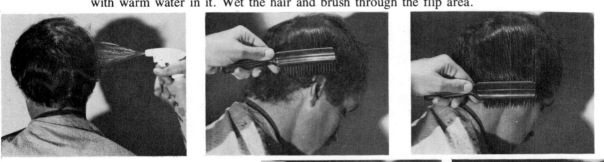

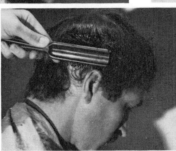

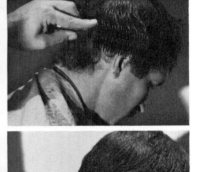

With the teeth of the brush
scraping the scalp, brush up
through the hair against the
hairgrain until it is
positioned over the flip area.
Roll the brush upward until
the teeth point away from the
scalp.

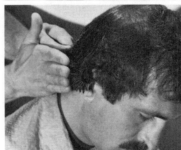

Place your free hand over the
teeth and continue rolling as
you pull the brush down and
out of the hair. This method
coaxes the hair ends to curve
inward and lie toward the
scalp. Let the hair air-dry
in this position and the
flips should be gone.

There are some situations where no amount of "de-flipping" will take
care of those stubborn flips:
1. **Protruding Ears**. The hair that comes over the ears will flip
out from the head when ears protrude far enough from the head, and you
have not left the hair long enough. This condition affects your
decision about the right length to leave the hair during the bulk-
cutting—the next chapter describes the remedy.
2. **The Nature of the Hair**. A lot of folks (mainly men) want their
curly hair to be straight. You could spend an eternity trying to
de-flip curly hair and it will still curl. Cutting curly hair to a
length of 3/4 – 1 inch usually has it lying into waves. If a longer
length is preferred, flippy curls are the rule: then **acceptance**
is the healthy solution—hair straightner is the alternative.

3. **Hairgrain Problem Areas**. A severe hairgrain clash can cause flippiness; the most common example of this occurs with the ducktail neckline. On a small percentage of folks, you'll find it doesn't matter what length you leave the hair, that stubborn neck hair flips out—it's rare, but you're likely to run across it. Again, acceptance is the only remedy. Another, more rare kind of clash can "pop up" on the top front hairline: a cowlick in this area may need a little extra hair length so the hair can bend a little and lie down. More specific information on these subjects is found in the next chapter.

4. **Hair Left Too Long**. A common flippy condition occurs when Type 2 hairgrain combines with fine-textured hair. If this hair is left too long, gravity and the hair's excess weight force the side hair to bend downward, instead of toward the back as the hairgrain would like it to lie. Whenever hair doesn't lie the way it wants to, you'll have flippy hair. The remedy is simple: cut it shorter.

6.12 PARTING THE HAIR

These rules only apply to straight and wavy hair—curlier hairtypes, with their out and away from the scalp way of being, don't lend themselves to a definite part as do the straighter varieties.

A. The Natural Part
Finding the natural part when you have given an equal-length cutting to the top hair is a simple procedure.

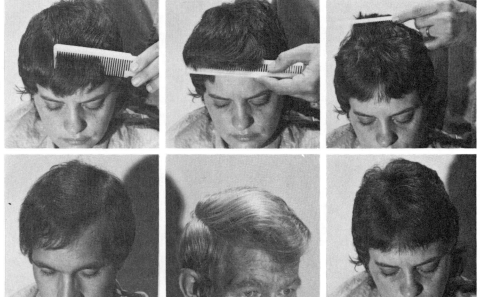

Comb all of the top hair toward the front. Then start at the front hairline and comb straight back to the crown region.

As the hair flops back toward the front, it will lie off to one side or the other, or it may split in the middle, revealing a center part.

This procedure is best done to hair that has been drum-dried so that no drying set has influenced the way the hair wants to lie. The equal-length cutting on top is mandatory for finding the natural part because it lets the hair lie as it wants—uneven cutting or the hair left longer on one side of the top hair than the other will have an influence on the way the hair lies.

On some heads of hair the top flops straight back toward the front. Hair like this, usually with a Type 1 hairgrain and the cowlick located at the center of the crown region, does not have a natural part, but it normally lends itself to the next way to part hair.

B. Forced Parting

To part a head of hair that does not have a natural part, you need to perform the following tool-handling procedure.

● Comb the hair forward, from the cowlick to the front hairline. Assuming a center cowlick, there are any number of different paths the comb can take through the hair.

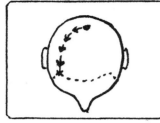
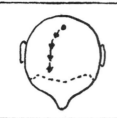
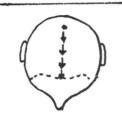
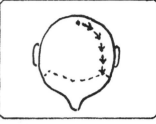

● Place the comb in a "comb line" created from the first step. This line must begin in the center of the cowlick, otherwise the cowlick stands on end like a rooster's tail.

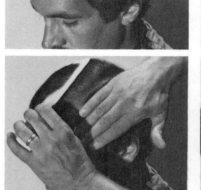

● Comb the top hair over the top toward the opposite side as you place your other hand over the side hair. Then hold the top hair with your free hand while you comb the hair below the part down the side.

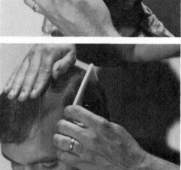

Forced parting has more rules:

(1) If the cowlick is on the side of the crown region, the hair should be parted on the same side that the cowlick is on. This makes for easier parting and it results in the hair lying according to the grain in almost all cases. The exception is the reverse hairgrain described back on page 6 of the first chapter: this unusual growth pattern needs to have the hair parted on the side of the head that is opposite of the cowlick. Here, you start the part at the cowlick, have it go **around the back of the head**, and then forward on the other side.

(2) If the cowlick is in the center of the crown region, check to see if the front hair wants to lie toward the left or right—use the hairgrain checkout explained in the first chapter. Or you can figure it out by looking for the "big puff": look closely at how much the hair stands out when it is combed first to one side and then to the other.

For example, if the hair is combed in this direction:

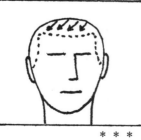

and the hair lies this way:

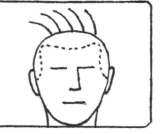

* * *

Inflation is when you pay $5.00 for the $2.00 haircut you use to get for $1.00 when you had hair.

Franklin P. Jones

Then the hair is combed in the opposite direction and it lies this way:

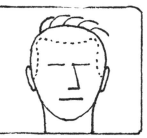

The lie of the hair **tells** you this last combing approach is the way the hair wants to lie—the hair is lying according to the hairgrain because it lies closer to the head. In this case, the hair would be parted on the right side of the person's head.

If no big puff is created when the hair is combed in either direction, then the hair can be parted on either side.

(3) The part should always be somewhere between the two "V"'s on the front hairline.

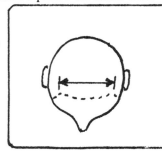

If you were to part the hair lower down into the side hair, you're battling the hairgrain and gravity. That side hair wants to lie in a downward direction; it would have to be bent to go over the top of the head, plus, it's always inclined to go back to its downward lying preference.

(4) If you have a cowlick on the front hairline, the part should be made into the center of it. Usually, the hair will "fall" into this kind of part by itself. Any other placement of the part would fight the hairgrain and have little chance for the hair to lie well.

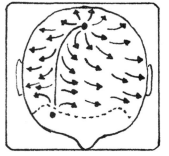

6.13 FINAL LOOKOVER AND MAKING ADJUSTMENTS

With the hair dried and brushed out you'll be able to see how well the "shingles are lying on the roof". This is when you give the hair a good looking over to see if any last minute corrections are needed. Put some distance (8 – 10 feet) between you and your efforts, and inspect. Ask yourself the following questions:

(1) Are the two sideburns the same length in relation to the ears on both sides? You have to raise up the longer side to match the shorter.

(2) Is the hair that comes over the ears cut to the same position on both sides? If your edge-cutting has left one ear more exposed than the other, trim the longer side to match the shorter.

(3) Are there any sloping edgelines? Check it all the way around, but give extra attention to the bangs and neckline. Trim as needed.

(4) Are there any heavy spots in your bulk-cutting? If there is an area that appears heavier than the rest, that heavy spot is caused by hair that is too long. It will need a little trimming to make it blend with the neighboring hair.

The longer hair that produces a heavy spot shows up in a couple of ways—as a bulky spot or a line. In either case, you need to go back through that area and use the same HGH position that was used during the bulk-removal.

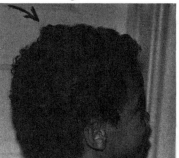

Bulky spot.

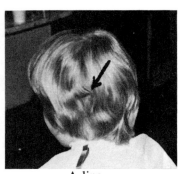

A line.

Where you comb out the hair—to get the longer hairs standing out from the head for the necessary smoothing off cuts—depends on the kind of hair you're cutting.

● If you are working on curly or kinky hair, its stand-out-from-the-head nature means the unevenness you see is the place where you comb out the hair.

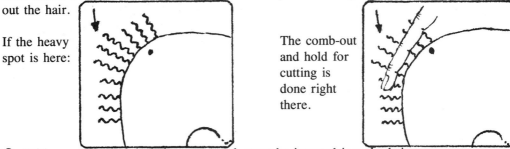

If the heavy spot is here:

The comb-out and hold for cutting is done right there.

● With wavy or straight hair, your comb must be inserted into the hair at some distance from where you see the line or heavy spot. The reasons for this are: (1) Straighter hair doesn't spring out from the head the way curlier hair does, **it lies down**, so the ends that cause the heavy spots are at some distance from their roots. (2) To get the hair to stand straight out from the scalp, you always have to start your comb-out at the roots of the hair you want to stand out.

For example, you give a 2 1/2 inch equal-length cut to a person with straight hair, and you find a bulky (uneven) spot.

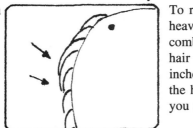

To remove this heavy spot, comb out the hair 1 – 2 inches above the heaviness you see.

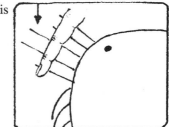

If the line or heavy spot is on the top of the head, your comb-out must be done some distance back toward the crown region.

Whatever hairtype you are working on, always comb up and hold some of the neighboring, correctly-cut hair to use as guide-hair. Be sure you don't cut any of those helping hairs.

6.14 CUTTING THOSE EXTRA, UNWANTED HAIRS

While women don't usually have problems with this, post-adolescent males have hairloss where they would like to keep it, and they grow it in a number of places where they could do without. Maybe it's Mother Nature's way of keeping things in balance?

A. Eyebrow Trimming

Here you need to learn a new way of using hands and tools, called the scissors-over-comb method. It's also used for beard trimming (see that section in the last chapter for more how-to) and it can be used with short, full haircuts—anywhere you want the hair extra short. Here the comb takes the place of the holding-guide-hand as a spacer tool. Like the HGH, the comb also has the function of holding the hair straight out from the skin for the cutting. In order to achieve this last function, the comb must move through the hair against or at least sideways to the hairgrain (if the comb moves through the hair in the same direction as the grain, the hair is combed down). When the comb moves the correct way, the hair builds up and stands out from the skin **at the backbar** of the comb: this is where you will do the cutting. Before you can snip the brows, you have know about their hairgrain.

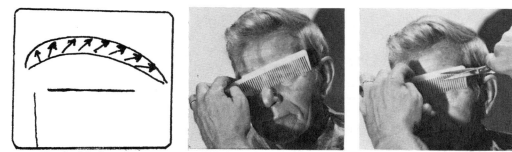

| Typical hairgrain. | HGH positions comb. | Cut protruding hairs. |

If you want to leave the brows longer, position the comb as shown, then move the comb away from the skin to the desired distance, and make your cuts.

B. The Ears

Hair usually crops out on the top edge of the ear and on the little "nubby" located at the front, center part of the ear.. This hair can be cut by using an electric razor, a safety razor and soap, or a scissors with the finger-bracing method.

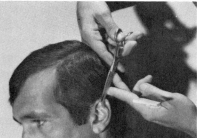

When you used this method for edge-cutting, you held the cutters perpendicular to the skin; here you hold the scissors at a 45 degree angle (or less) to cut those hairs as short as possible. Always be sure there isn't any skin between the blades—go slowly!

C. Nose Hair

If there is such a thing as "unsightly" hair, it has to be a clump of hairs protruding out of the nose! Use the finger-bracing method to cut **only** those hairs that protrude. Never do any cutting inside of the nostril—lots of potential for trouble there. If there are any hairs growing on top of the nose, trim those off too.

D. Stray Hairs on the Sides of the Neck and Below the Neckline

Use a razor, preferably a safety razor with soap or shaving lather, to remove the extra hairs that grow beyond the edge-cutting line. Or you can use the scissors-over-comb method that was used to trim eyebrows. This approach, like cutting the brows, leaves the hair cut to a length that is equal to, or a little longer than the thickness of the comb if the comb is held so it touches the skin. If a longer length is desired, hold the comb at some distance from the skin while cutting.

6.15 SAFETY CONSIDERATIONS

Safety is free: it only costs a little time and concern. Be extra generous with it.

A. Relatively Safe Situations

When your cutting is done with the holding-guide-hand (HGH) holding the hair, you have a fairly safe working situation. The only time you have to be concerned is when you move your thumb in and out of the thumb grip—the thumb blade might flop open if the pivot screw is to loose (see pages 51 and 52).

B. Extra Care Situations

When you edge cut, your scissors work close to the skin. Until you are comfortable and experienced with this kind of cutting, go slowly and always be aware of where the points of the blades are.

● When using the finger-bracing method, be sure to hold the blades at a 90 degree angle to the skin, and keep the back of the thumb blade in contact with the skin. Don't be in a hurry with this way of cutting.

● The scissors-and-comb method needs extra care because you won't have anything for the scissors to rest on while its being positioned, or when cutting. Use the pivot movement with the comb for extra working room, and go slow.

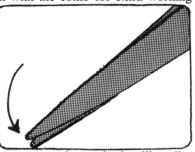

● Never work with scissors if the points of the blades overlap.

● Don't attempt to give a haircut to someone who can't sit still until you're an experienced haircutter—you have enough to deal with without having to dodge a person's sudden movements. (The last chapter tells how to get maximum cooperation when cutting children's hair.)

● Watch out for ears. This applies to all the edging methods, but especially the fingers-bracing method. I have only snipped a person's ear once in my haircutting career, but that was one time too many. I paid close attention to the points of the blades while edging around the ears on a short haircut—the center of the blades spoiled my day.

C. Miscellaneous Safety Tips

● Earrings. If your haircuttee is wearing earrings that can get snagged by the comb, be sure they are taken off before you begin.

● Warts and moles. These little growths need extra accomodation on your part. If a wart or mole is on the scalp, I start my bulk-removal in that area, so the comb doesn't bump into it as I'm working through the paths—it's hard to keep them in mind while striving for smooth cutting. If the growth is on the neck it needs special handling if you shave the extra neck hairs: blot the lather off before you begin.

● As a beginner, the way to avoid any mishap is to concentrate on what you're doing and work in a slow, deliberate manner. To this end, you should refrain from conversation while cutting hair: at least, keep it to a bare minimum. Besides the safety factor, this rule-of-thumb is important from the standpoint of quality cutting. I have had many customers who like to talk while getting their hair cut—unless I'm giving an extra easy haircut that doesn't require my complete concentration, I'll explain that I can give a good haircut or I can carry on a good conversation, but I can't do both at the same time. Both keep the mind busy. The professional haircutters I've worked with who were strong on chatter always produced something less than quality haircuts, and they were the ones who had problems with safety.

As far as the development of tool handling skills, you now have all it takes to achieve the goal of a precision haircut. The haircut chapters show specialized uses for these skills such as sideburn trimming, tapering, and more. Before we begin our cut-by-cut how-to, you'll learn about length and shape decisions.

* * *

Don't talk unless you can improve the silence.   Vermont proverb

7 DETERMINING THE RIGHT LENGTH

7.1 TWO PARTS TO A WELL-DONE HAIRCUT

These scissors and comb haircuts produce hair that not only stays in shape no matter what happens to it, they need the smallest investment in time, money, resource use, and concern. To achieve these positive results, two ingredients are essential to your success.

1. **Cut the Hair Evenly** Whichever of the three haircuts you give, you will cut the hair so that it lies like shingles-on-a-roof. The tool handling skills you've learned and the cut-by-cut haircut chapters assures your cutting is even and precise.

2. **Cut the Hair to the Right Length** You could do an outstanding job of cutting the hair evenly, but if the hair is cut to the wrong length, it's a sorry haircut. There are several factors that affect your decision about the right length for any person's hair.

- What hairtype are you working with?
- What is the texture of the hair?
- What, if any, special hair problems does the person have?
- What does your haircuttee prefer?

You have to take into consideration all of these factors to answer the question: How long should I leave the hair?

7.2 CUTTING OFF EXCESS LENGTH MAKES HAIR CAREFREE

For low maintenance hairstyles that only need a shampoo and towel-dry every day or two, you must cut off the **unnecessary** hair length, and leave the hair just long enough to lie well. This rule-of-thumb applies primarily to the hair on top of the head: it is here that hair gets heavy and bulky and hard to manage—if you have a big mop on top, wash-and-wear haircare is difficult at best.

Your hair-length determinations are mainly concerned with the top hair. At least 90 percent of the time, sides and back hair can be cut to any length and shape—provided, of course, it blends-in with the top hair. Exceptions to this rule are pointed out in section 6.

7.3 HAIRTYPE MAKES A BIG DIFFERENCE

You can easily decide about length for wavier, curly, and kinky types of hair: they offer complete flexibility as to length and shape. In addition, these kinds of hair are generally not affected by the hair problems discussed later. Because these hairtypes tend to be thick and heavy if left too long on top, most people prefer a length of 1 1/2 – 2 1/2 inches on the topside. The shorter the cutting, the straighter or wavier the hair lies; the longer the length, the curlier the hair.

Straight and slightly wavy hair are the hairtypes that present problems. Cut them too short and they won't lie down; leave them too long and they become floppy mops that never keep a good shape. These kinds of hair are usually the ones that may have one or more of the special hair problems discussed later. They may also have limitations as to the kind of haircut that can be given. For straighter hair, the next hair factor is the crucial one.

7.4 HAIR TEXTURE

The diameter of a hair makes no difference on wavier, curly, or kinky hair. With straight or slightly wavy hair, this is the factor that determines the best length to leave the hair. The rule is: the finer the hair, the shorter it should be cut; the coarser the hair, the longer you should leave it. These general guidelines for bulk-removal length, leaves straight hair lying its **best**.

TEXTURE/LENGTH GUIDELINES

Fine hair	1 – 2 inches
Medium hair	1 1/2 – 2 1/2 inches
Coarse hair	2 – 3 inches or more

Most of my equal-length haircuts are 2 – 2 1/2 inches long—this leaves half the ear covered after the edging is done.

7.5 TEXTURE/LENGTH TEST FOR STRAIGHT HAIR

If you're unsure about the texture of the hair to be cut, this test can be used. First, yank out or cut off one top hair at the scalp. Hold it at the root end, as close to the very end as possible, and straight up. Keep cutting it shorter until you have the kind of bend shown in the second drawing.

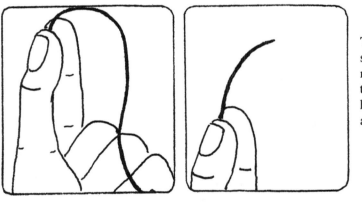

The next step is to measure the cut hair with a ruler.

Then you need to take a close-up look at the top hair to see at what angle the hair grows from the scalp. If the person has a 1 in a 100 kind of hair that grows straight up (90-degrees) from the scalp, the measurement you got with the ruler is the length the hair should be cut. If the hair grows out at a more common 45-degree angle, you would subtract 1 inch from the ruler's measurement. A 65 to 70-degree grow-out would need a 1/2 inch subtracted from the measurement.

If the hair is thinning on top, cut it 1/2 – 3/4 inch shorter than the length you calculated from the texture test. Thinning hair tends to lie close to the head because it does not have much neighborly support. Those sparse top hairs have more fullness if cut shorter.

7.6 SPECIAL HAIR PROBLEMS THAT AFFECT LENGTH AND SHAPE

Some heads of hair have conditions making it mandatory that the hair is cut to a particular length or shape, and you might even need to limit yourself to one kind of haircut. With most haircuttees there won't be any problems, but you don't know unless you look closely at the hair. You avoid unhappy results by doing a close inspection and figuring these possible problems into your hair-length determinations.

A. Short Growing Hair Around the Bottom of the Sides

About 10 percent of men have this condition. No cause is known, nor can anything be done to change it. This stunted hairgrowth looks much like the fellow's beard hair—how it creeps up into the longer growing hair around the sides is a question without an answer. You as a haircutter have to deal with it, however, it doesn't really become a problem that affects your haircutting unless this condition exists more than 3/4 – 1 inch above the bottom hairline.

<u>Remedy</u> More than a question of hair length, this problem has to be dealt with in terms of which of the three basic haircuts should be given? When 1 – 2 inches of the lower hair is affected, you will find that equal-length shaping doesn't work too well. Instead of the hair lying smoothly around the edges, it wants to be flippy and the hair won't reach down to the normal length on the ears.

Here is how it appears with a 2 inch equal-length cut.

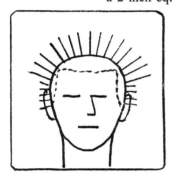
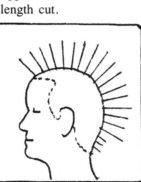
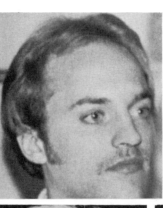
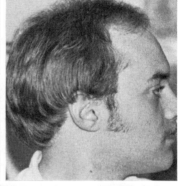

A long, layered cut covers over this problem fairly well. However, the hair doesn't even reach the bottom of the ears, and it tends to flip around the edges, (but less than the equal-length cut).

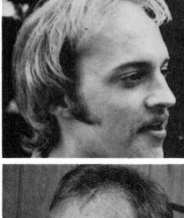
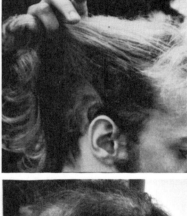

The best choice for a good fitting shape is the short, full cut. All the hairs blend together—no longer hairs cover over the shorter hairs. While this cut produces the best fit, there are some who don't like their hair cut this short.

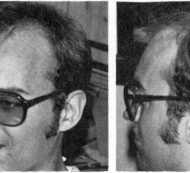

With the haircut limitations this problem presents, I suggest you avoid working on someone with this condition until you have enough experience to handle the more advanced haircuts.

B. Protruding Ears

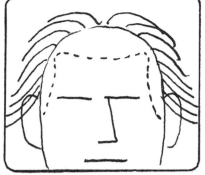

When the tops of the ears protrude 3/4 inch or more from the head, the hair that covers them usually flips out if cut too short: it looks like wings on the sides of the head.

If the hairline above the ears is close to the top of the ear, the problem is worse. If there is 1/2 inch or more distance between the ear and the hairline above, the problem isn't as severe. You will find this condition on 5 – 10 percent of your haircuttees.

<u>Remedy</u> There are only two good ways to deal with this problem.

● Leave the hair on the sides long enough (2 1/2 inches or more) during the bulk-removal, so half or more of the ear is covered after you have done the final edging. This only works well if the texture of the hair allows that kind of longer length. If the hair has a fine texture, you are better off with the next option.

● Give an extra full, short cut with the hair cut above the ears. Extra fullness around the sides minimizes the visual effect of protruding ears, and the hair won't flip out. Because the short, full cut requires quite a bit of haircutting experience, as a beginner you should choose the first option, even if the hair is fine.

C. Double Cowlick

When you have two cowlicks in the crown region, you **may** have hair that stands out from the head if cut too short.

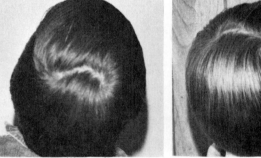
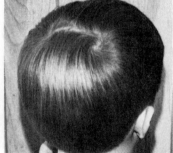

The area between the cowlicks is where the rooster's tail wants to stand on end. Only 10 – 15 percent of double cowlicks need extra length on top to avoid hairs standing on end. The difficult ones have straight, coarse-textured hair, with the two cowlicks within 1 1/2 inches of each other.

<u>Remedy</u> If the hair is as described above, you will need an extra inch or more of length on the upper part of the head. Use the texture/length test to help decide the length that allows the hair to lie down. Here you will need to go with the length the ruler tells you—don't subtract from the measurement. I can't recall ever leaving the top hair longer than 3 1/2 inches; usually, 3 inches is plenty of length for the hair to bend into a lying position.

The extra length on top may leave the bangs too long. Make your edge cuts there shorter than the normal, minimum cutting approach.

D. Low Cowlick

A cowlick in a lower-than-normal position can produce another rooster tail condition (pages 8 and 9 in the first chapter described this). The reason for this stand-out hair is quite different from a double cowlick, and the cure is exactly the opposite. This problems pops up on about 5 percent of the population.

<u>Remedy</u> To overcome the hair's battle with the forces of gravity, you need to cut it short enough so it won't bend. This can be done in

* * *

A problem well stated is a problem half solved.   Charles F. Kettering one of two ways on equal-length or short, full haircuts.

(1) Determine the best length for the hair, then proceed to cut the hair 1/2 - 3/4 inch shorter than your best guess. For example, if you decided on 2 inches, change that to 1 1/2 inches or a little shorter.

(2) After all the bulk-removal is cut to the determined length, go back to the cowlick region for some more cutting. You concentrate your re-cutting on a 3 - 4 inch wide circle with the cowlick in the center. As you work through this area, (two paths should do it,) gradually grasp the hair shorter as you approach the cowlick, and then gradually longer—to the normal HGH position—as you move away from the cowlick. This amounts to a 1/2 - 3/4 inch deep "sink-hole" in the haircut.

If you're giving one of the long haircuts to someone with a low cowlick, the above solutions can only be applied to the "umbrella" way of shaping, or the shorter versions of the "combination cut'. The regular version of the long, layered cut has enough length in the crown region for the hair to comfortably bend into a lying position.

While the haircuts taught here normally keep a good shape for a couple of months or so, hair with a low cowlick usually needs cutting once every month or less to keep it from standing out.

E. Ducktail Neckline

Necklines that appear like a duck's tail have caused many folks much frustration, expense, and time wasted in efforts to tame down that unruly neck hair. It doesn't lie the way they like, and as it grows longer it starts doing flippy, contrary kinds of things. Nothing can be done to change this condition, but there are effective ways to deal with it. This problem ranges from slight to severe.

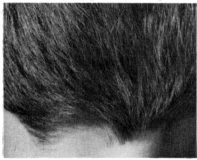

Slight.

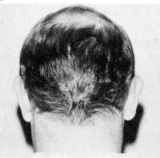

Moderate.

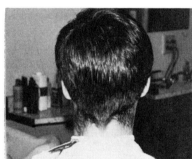

Severe.

Usually the tail is in the middle as shown above, but it can be off to one side or the other.

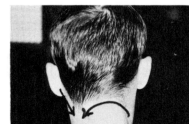

These photos all show this curvy hairgrain phenomenon with short hair so it can be easily seen. Longer hair hides this condition to some extent, but long hair and a ducktail usually adds up to flippy hair at the neckline.

<u>Remedy</u> In the big majority of cases, the ducktail neckline does not require any special shaping or length modifications—you can cut as if it were not there. However, when moderate to severe ducktails combine with coarse, straight hair, you have to change your ordinary methods. There are a couple of ways to deal with problem ducktails.

(1) Cut it extra short. An equal-length cut with the neck-area hair tapered shorter is usually effective, but you may have to give a short, full haircut to get it short enough. In an extreme case, you would use the scissors-over-comb way to cut the hair in the lower neck area. (See the beard trimming section in the last chapter for more on

this shortest cutting method.)
(2) Leave it extra long. The long, layered cut or the longest version
of the equal-length cut or shaping the neck hair so it has an
increasing length (see the next chapter, section 5-B) leaves the hair
long enough to bend over and cover this condition. While this remedy
might leave the hair flippy at the neckline, any length between the
short and long remedies has problem ducktails standing on end.

Handcombing is **always** a good, relaxed way to groom hair with
the haircuts you are learning, but if there ever was a hair condition
that **needs** this hand-done approach, it's hair with a ducktail
neckline. If the rest of the head of hair has an every-hair-in-place
type of grooming, the somewhat out-of-place hairs in the neck area
will stand out from the rest of the hair like a sore thumb. Handcombing helps to blend all the hair together.

F. Cowlick on the Top, Front Hairline
This cowlick condition, found on 5 – 10 percent
of people, normally isn't located in the hair—
if you look extra close, you'll see the cowlick
center in the peach fuzz on the forehead.

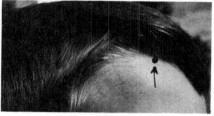

While the cowlick's center is not in the hair, that front hairline is
affected by the hairgrain this cowlick establishes.
Remedy This hairgrain condition is not much of a problem as long
as you **go with** the way the hair wants to lie. When you try to
force the bangs to lie in a direction that is contrary to the hair's
natural preferences, you need extra length on top. On rare heads this
kind of cowlick needs extra length even if you allow the hair to lie
the way it wants. There are two ways to provide this extra length:
(1) Cut the top section about one inch longer than you normally would.
(2) Leave the front 1 1/2 – 2 inches of hair—behind the top, front
hairline—with a gradually increasing length. (This cutting technique
is shown in the next chapter, pages 117 and 118.)

1 in 1,000 heads of hair have a front cowlick that is a 1/2 – 1
inch behind the front hairline. This rare condition **always** needs
extra length to lie well, usually more than that suggested above.

7.7 WHAT THE HAIRCUTTEE WANTS

The last consideration in your efforts to determine the best length
and shape for the hair is the preference of the person who receives
your haircut. To deal with this, you must first look over their hair,
then ask questions, offer suggestions, and be a good listener.

Haircut communication must be clear and concise, but of course,
this is easier said than done. Ignorance, hair myths, and the wrong
choice of words can muddle-up this need for clarity.
● **Are they knowledgeable?** Hair type, texture, and special problems
prevent many options—you may have to spend time educating beforehand.
● **The bending trap**. Do they want a hairstyle that requires
constant bending with comb or brush, hair dryer or curling iron. Point
out the hassle involved and how much damage is caused by this approach
to hair before you leave the hair with extra length so it can bend.
● **Heavy hair**. Many folks unknowingly request to have their hair
"thinned-out." They don't necessarily mean they want the heavy top
hair thinned-out with thinning shears, they are just using an old term
to describe their desire to get rid of the hard to handle hair on top.

If they do want the use of those thinners, refer back to pages 21 and 22 for some education.

● **Descriptive terms**. In my efforts to find out how a person wants their hair cut, I usually ask how they like to wear the hair around the ears (the answer to this question tells me what bulk-removal length is needed). Watch out for the term ''over the ears': for some, they mean **above** the ears, for others, they mean **covering** the ears. You have to take what they say, then put it into your own words and ask them if that is what they mean?

● **Cutting hair from a picture**. Occasionally a person brings along a picture of someone and says: I want it cut like this. Bad idea! Rarely will your haircuttee's hair characteristics match those of the person in the picture. This expression of hair desires is a useful point of departure: you can use that picture to explain how the wishful haircuttee's head of hair is different, how that difference results in a different appearance, and what other options are open.

Meeting your haircuttee's desires might require some give-and-take: on the basis of what you **now** know about hair and what they desire, a little compromise maybe necessary. If they want you to ignore what you've learned, do yourself a favor and send them to a pro—you don't need to start your haircutting efforts with unhappy results. I can't say you'll **always** be right on the basis of the information in this chapter, but you will be able to make **educated judgements** worth following. If your length calculations are off the mark, **they won't be far off**! When your best guess is a little off, that doesn't mean you have produced a poor haircut: it only means you have some room for improvement on the second cutting. Using the haircut record system described in the last chapter will help insure you've learned from the first haircut, and improvements are made on the second.

7.8 HAIR THINGS THAT ARE IMPORTANT TO MOST PEOPLE

Many people have a tried-and-true knowledge about what works best on their hair. Besides smoothly-cut hair that lies well and the kind of basic overall shaping given to the hair, past experience has people concerned with particular parts of the haircut. This list is arranged in order of importance, but it's strictly an individual matter—the last thing listed here can be the big concern for your haircuttee.

1. **The Length Around the Ears**. How far the hair comes down over the ear on an equal-length cut seems to be the big one for most people. Keep in mind that the length you leave the hair during bulk-cutting determines the length of the hair covering the ear (see page 76). Also remember your final edging will raise the bottom edge about 1/2 inch or a little more, and be sure to take into account the shrinking edgeline factors explained in chapter 6, section 6.

2. **Having the Hair Feather-Back**. Since the early 1970s, more and more folks have begun wearing their hair back off the face. All three haircuts, especially the equal-length cut, can be worn this way, but it depends largely on having a Type 2 hairgrain. If you have a Type 1 grain, the hair must be left at least 1 inch longer than normal to have it bend toward the back. Because extra length creates heavy hang-down hair, yet extra length is needed to bend the hair, this is one haircuttee's preference that sometimes can't be satisfied.

3. **The Bangs**. Back in the 1960s and early 1970s, the length of the bangs was quite a big thing. The recent trend to the feathered-back approach changed this. Before it was a matter of how much forehead

showed, now the idea is to get the bangs hair to lie back, off to the sides or top hair. Times change, but cutting the bangs so they don't block one's vision is still a concern. Page 76 tells how the bulk-removal length determines the length of bangs.

4. **Top Hair**. When the top hair has too much length, it becomes heavy hair that lies flat on the head. Many people use this as their reminder that it's time for another haircut. The three basic haircuts in this book are designed for maximum body and fullness on top.

5. **Neck Hair Length**. How long or short the hair is at the neckline is a big stickler to many. For some it's bothersome; some have a masculine (no flips) versus feminine (hooray for flips) thing about it. The next chapter shows how to make modifications on the neck hair.

Always ask your haircuttees what their haircut ''quirks'' are, and what past problems they have had with their hair and haircuts. The idea is to accomodate them whenever possible.

7.9 MY TWO HAIRSTYLING RULES

If you've ever read books or magazine articles written by well-known hairstylists, you know about the endless prescriptions for how the hair should be cut and worn: a face with prominent cheekbones needs so and so; the triangular-shaped head must have the hair cut this way; the oblong face requires more hair here, and less hair there; the round face demands. . . . There are so many ''experts'' preaching different how-tos, you find contradictions all over the place. I have kept my hairstyling rules simple and consistent—these are my guidelines:

1. **Make the hair easy to care for and easy to ignore.**
2. **Cut the hair to fit the person's size.**

The first rule is always achievable if the person wants an unburdened head of hair. All three haircuts should be cut so the top hair and the rest of the hair have all the excess length removed—the hair is left just long enough so it lies well. When you leave only the essential hair length, you have created low maintenance, ignorable hair.

The second rule depends on the hair I have to work with. There are some heads of hair—especially straight, fine hair or hair with special problems—that don't lend themselves to hair length or shape options. On the other hand, at least 75 percent of the time, the heads of hair I work on allow me all kinds of choices. If the hair presents limitations, I work within those limits. If the hair gives me choices, I recommend a length and shape that balances the hair with the person's physical size. These are some examples.

● If you have a tall person, cut the hair on the longer side. A shorter person would get a shorter haircut.

● For a long neck, leave the neck hair longer. A short forehead gets a shorter bulk-cutting on top, so the bangs are also shorter.

● Long sideburns fit a man with a long face, and vice versa.

This rule of fit and balance and the above examples are not chiseled in stone. I give haircuts to some folks and the opposite of what is suggested here works well. It is all a matter of personal preference, but if I'm asked for advice, I know this approach brings the hair into harmony with a person's overall physical makeup.

You now have all the ingredients it takes to get extra good results on your first attempt at precision haircutting—**GOOD FOR YOU!**

* * *

Great things are done on purpose for a purpose.   Anonymous

8.1 INTRODUCTION

You begin by learning the haircut that proves there is **BEAUTY IN SIMPLICITY** in the endless ways of having hair cut. The uncomplicated nature of this cut makes it the easiest haircut to learn: just pull the hair straight out from the head, all over, and cut it to the same length. This basic shingles-on-a-roof haircut produces a head of hair that always keeps a good shape with the least amount of haircare.

As a beginner, you will find this to be the best possible haircut to start with because it also happens to be the most popular way to wear the hair. The popularity of this cut goes back many generations: it has been called the layered cut, the windblown, the afro or fro, the feathered cut, the radial cut, the inch-cut, the three-inch cut—whatever its name, you are talking about a **basic** way to have hair cut that a majority of people prefer.

The name equal-length cut implies a sameness in appearance from one haircut to the next: don't be misled. You could give ten of these haircuts to ten people—the final appearance of each would be quite different. The following contribute to each haircut's uniqueness:
1. **Hair Factors**. Hair type, hairgrain, hair texture, and thickness or thinness combine to make every equal-length cut appear different.
2. **Haircut Factors**. The equal-length cut lends itself to different cutting lengths: as short as one inch or less on finer-textured or curlier types of hair, or as long as four or more inches (not recommended for a beginner's efforts). In addition, this chapter teaches some easy shaping variations that leave some parts of the hair longer or shorter than the overall equal-length approach.
3. **The Human Factor**. Haircutting is a hand craft. When you produce things by hand, the results always vary a little from one effort to the next—it has that one-of-a-kind quality called character.

These before-and-after pictures show this haircut's uniqueness:

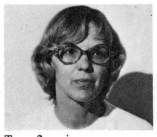

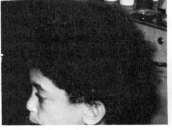
Cut to 2 1/2 inches all over.

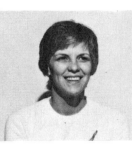

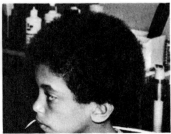
Cut to 2 inches, and slightly tapered in back.

Type 2 grain.
Medium,
straight hair.

Type 2 grain.
Coarse, curly
to kinky hair.

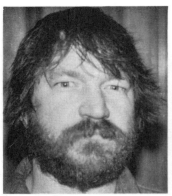

Type 1, fine to
medium texture.
Slight waviness.

Cut to 1 3/4
inches, and
tapered in back.

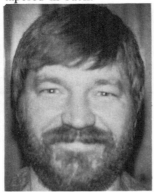

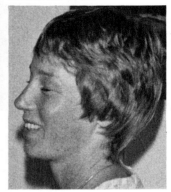

Cross between Type
1 and 2. Fine to
medium texture.
Straight hair with
protruding ears.

Cut to 2 1/2
inches all over.

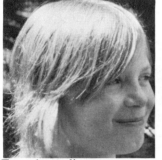

Type 1, medium,
straight hair.

Cut to 2 inches
and tapered back.

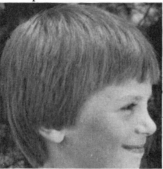

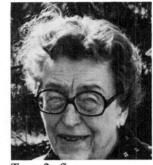

Type 2, fine,
wavy hair with
double cowlick.

Cut to 3 inches,
bottom of sides
little shorter.

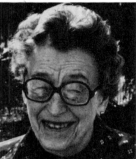

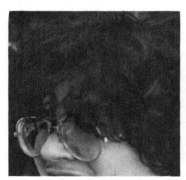

Type 2, coarse,
wavy hair.

Cut to 3 inches,
tapered to 1 1/2
inches in back.

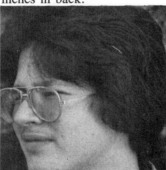

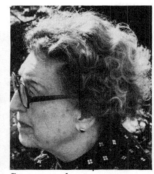

Same as above.

Back tapered to
1 inch length.

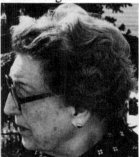

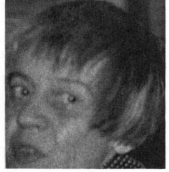

Type 1, extra fine,
straight hair.
Low cowlick.

Cut to 2 inches.
Cowlick area is
1 1/2 inches.

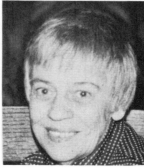

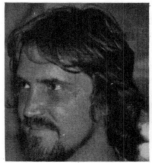

Type 1, medium,
straight hair.
Protruding ears.

Cut to 2 1/2
inches. Bangs
and neckline a
little shorter.

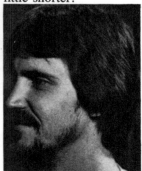

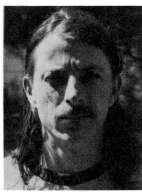

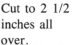

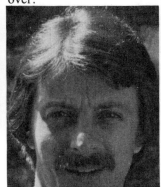

Cut to 2 1/2 inches all over.

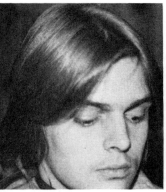

Type 2, medium to coarse, straight hair.

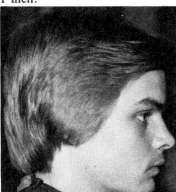

Cut to 3 inches, back tapered to 1 inch.

Cross between Type 1 and 2. Medium texture, straight hair.

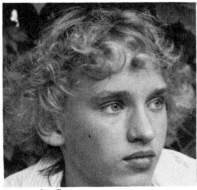

Type 2, fine to medium, wavy hair. Protruding ears.

Cut to 2 1/2 inches. Back tapered to 1 1/2 inches.

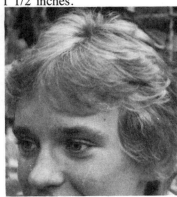

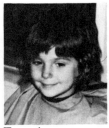

Type 1, straight to slightly wavy, fine hair.

Cut to little less than 2 inches—back has increasing length.

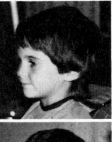

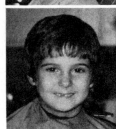

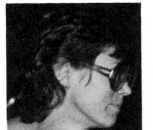

Type 2, medium, straight hair.

Cut to 2 inches, increasing length in back.

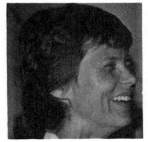

Cut to 2 inches all over.

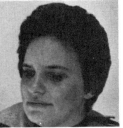

Cross between Type 1 and 2, straight, fine to medium hair. Double cowlick, but extra length is not needed.

Cut to 2 inches, back is tapered to 1 inch.

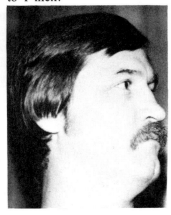

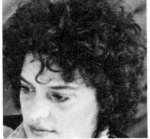

Type 2, medium, extra wavy hair.

After looking at these examples of equal-length haircuts, perhaps you're wondering what to expect from your efforts? To start with, a warning to perfectionists: do yourself a favor and give the book to someone not burdened by faultless standards—cutting 100,000 hairs will only leave you frustrated! For you who can accept less-than-perfect results, you'll learn how to give quality haircuts that are better than what the average professional gives. To explain this, you have to know about the world of professional cutters:

(1) About a third of the pros do excellent work that fully meets their patron's needs. They produce precision cuts on a consistent basis.

(2) Another third get "so-so" results. Sometimes you receive a good cut, sometimes it's poor. They may suffer from job burn-out, or perhaps they are more interested in conversation or in selling you extra services and products. There are many things to take one's mind off haircutting, but a poor haircut results when the mind drifts off.

(3) The last third try to do the job, but they don't know what they are doing. These "hackers" should find another way to make a living.

You have important advantages on your side:

● You **care**! Wanting to do your best combined with an honest effort makes a very positive contribution to the results you get.

● You have 20 years of haircutting knowledge to guide you. This tried-and-true approach has you avoiding all manner of beginner's pitfalls.

● You don't have time pressures. You have ample time to analyze your haircuttee's hair and reach agreement on the haircut. The cutting is done when convenient and you'll take whatever time is needed to do the job right. A little change/correction can be made whenever you want.

● Your goal is healthy, easy-to-care-for hair. You could achieve an extra precise cutting on a haircut, but if the hair **must** have a lot of time or damaging extras in its daily maintenance, it's a sorry haircut. The haircuts you'll be giving makes it possible to practice a healthy, **less-is-better** way to care for hair.

Let's assume that somehow haircuts could be ranked on a 1 to 10 scale: number 1 would be a hairy disaster, and number 10 would be a perfectionist's dream. From my experience with beginners I can predict you'll start around the 7 level. With experience you'll slowly improve (with an occasional reversal) until you reach the 9 level I usually operate at. Just remember: you're not a machine that stamps out a consistent product time after time—you'll have your ups-and-downs. With the help of the haircut recording system described on page 181, you can learn from your downs and improve on them.

8.2 BULK-CUTTING OVERVIEW

To get from the first to the last cut in the bulk-removal, with every hair cut to the length you want, you must use a systematic sequence of sections, pathways, and cuts. This way of cutting hair is the same approach used when mowing a lawn. You don't cut grass with a "here a cut, there a cut" approach, nor do you take a wandering path all over the lawn: to get all of the lawn cut in the most effective way, you use a systematic approach that has paths cut beside already-cut paths.

A. The Sequence to Follow
When you follow this sequence of sections, pathways, and cuts within pathways, you will mow them off without a single "blade" being left uncut. You start on the top of the head.

* * *

Nobody can be perfect unless he admits his faults, but if he has faults how can he be perfect?   Dr. Laurence J. Peter

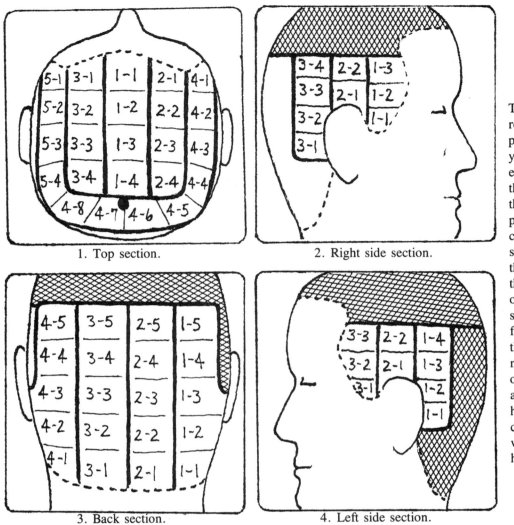

1. Top section.　　　　　　　2. Right side section.

3. Back section.　　　　　　　4. Left side section.

The numbers represent the pathways and cuts you make. For example, 1-1 in the top section is the first pathway's initial cut; 1-2 is the first path, second cut; 1-3 would be the first path, third cut. Moving on, 2-1 is the second path's first cut; 2-2 is the second path's next cut; and so on. The checkered areas show the hair that has been cut as you are working around the head.

B. Why Do It This Way?

● The methodical simplicity of this approach means you always know where you are, where you have been, and where you are going next.

● As you move from one cut to the next, your comb travels through the hair against, or at least sideways to the hairgrain. This is what is needed to get the hair combed out from its lying position.

● When you work on neighboring pathways, you are able to use the guide-hair aid. While there are a few areas where you can't make use of guide-hair, over 90 percent of your cuts have this help.

C. The Number of Paths and the Cuts Within a Path are Approximate

Always use the cutting sequence shown above, but keep in mind that the number of cuts in a pathway and the number of pathways in a section depend on such things as the size of the head, how thick (more cuts in a path) versus how thin (less cuts) the hair is, and the size of your holding-guide-hand (HGH). For example, I am able to use just 3 paths on the top section for some children, but, for an adult with a large head, I may have to add a couple of paths to get to the outside limits of the top section. On a smaller head, I may only need 3 cuts to get from the front to the back of the top section; a larger head will

* * *

There are many truths of which the full meaning cannot be realized until personal experience has brought it home.　　　　　John Stuart Mill probably take 5 or as many as 6 cuts.

The number of pathways or cuts within a path is not important—it is important to follow the **sequence** of sections, pathways, and cuts within the paths.

D. **One Cut for Each Inch of Travel Through a Pathway**
As you go through a pathway, you make one cut per inch of travel through the path. Assuming an average sized HGH, your cuts will be about 1 1/2 – 2 inches wide.

8.3 YOUR POSITION WHILE CUTTING

Pages 67 and 68 in chapter 5 described a couple of basic height positions that maximize your vision while cutting, and make tool handling easier. For the same reasons you also change **where** you stand during the haircut. To help simplify the description of where to stand while cutting the different pathways, we make reference to the hours of the clock.

Stand behind haircuttee and look down at the top of their head. Imagine the head is numbered like the face of a clock. The nose is 12 o'clock, and the other hours designate your other locations around the head.

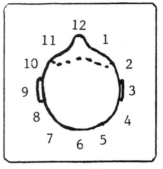

If I tell you to stand at a 6 o'clock position, stand directly behind the haircuttee; at 9 o'clock you stand to the haircuttee's left; at 4 – 5 o'clock stand at the right rear; 11 o'clock is a front left position.

8.4 BULK-REMOVAL: THE CUT-BY-CUT HOW-TO

As you do the bulk-cutting, you may find it works best to have your haircuttee read the directions aloud and show you the photos. The best alternative is to have the book opened on a table next to you.

Before you start, go back to page 46 in chapter 3, and be sure you have followed all the steps in "Preparations for Haircutting Success". Do the approximate cutting if needed, and you're ready to begin!

A. **Top Section**
You begin with pathway 1. Move from the front-top-center hairline straight back to the top center of the crown region. The 1 1/2 – 2 inch width of the path, and the one cut for each inch of travel back to the crown region is easy to work with; however, the width can be narrower or wider, depending on the size of your HGH.

Don't try to get too much hair between those holding fingers. Holding too much hair causes the kind of unevenness shown at the right. Thicker heads of hair are affected more by this overloading the hand problem.

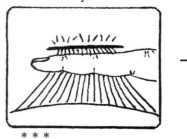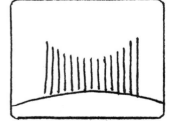

* * *

The smallest good deed is better than the grandest good intention.

Message on a poster at my dentist's office

The farther we get from ourselves, the closer we get to God. Anonymous

Some things have to be believed to be seen.   Ralph Hodgson

To get started, seat the haircuttee on a high stool or chair. You stand behind in a 6 o'clock position. Wet the hair thoroughly and comb it forward on top and down the sides and back. Rewet the hair as often as necessary during the haircut. If needed, use the helping-hand method shown on page 66 to get the hair combed up for the first cut.

Pathway 1 You may need to make more than 4 cuts if the hair is thick or the head is large. When you reach the top back of the head, comb the top hair forward again and go back through path 1 a second time. (You might not cut off any hair, but you will be sure this initial path is cut to the desired length in a nice, straight manner.)

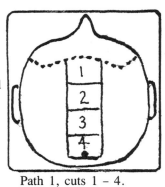

Path 1, cuts 1 – 4.

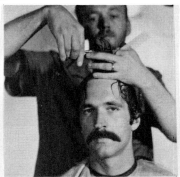

Cut 1.

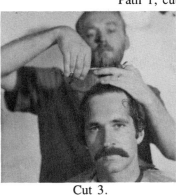

Cut 2.

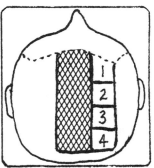

Cut 3.

Cut 4.

There is no guide-hair to use as an aid with this first path, so be extra sure your HGH produces a consistent length.

Pathway 2 In cutting path 2, you use the important guide-hair aid. Be sure to comb up some of that already-cut hair from path 1 while you work through path 2. Here the scissors point to the guide-hair at the "V" of the holding fingers.

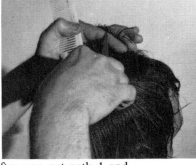

Remember to recomb the hair forward on top, after you cut path 1 and after each path on the top section. Use the helping-hand aid to get started on the first cut if needed, and whenever it's convenient on any of the rest of the pathways you make through the hair.

Continue at the 6 o'clock position. Remember to keep a pinching pressure between the holding fingers until the comb is reinserted in the hair after each hand-tool manipulation made in the path.

Path 2, cuts 1 – 4.

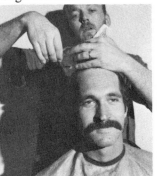

Cut 1.

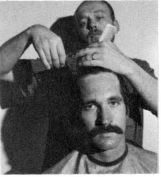

Cut 2.

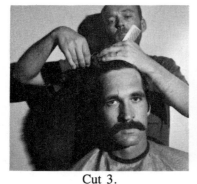

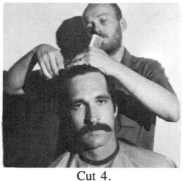

Cut 3.   Cut 4.

The guide-hair at the "V" of your holding fingers does not show in these photos, but it was there after careful comb and holding-hand manipulation.

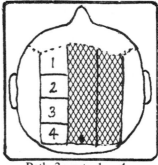

Path 3, cuts 1 – 4.

Pathway 3 This path requires the same 6 o'clock position. Here, the guide-hair shows at the tips of the holding fingers. Don't cut those already-cut hairs, just use them.

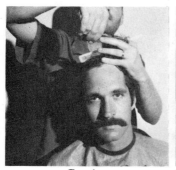

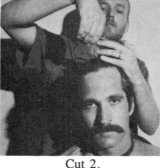

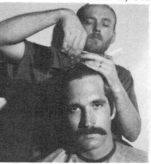

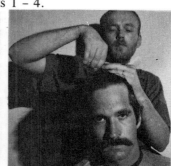

Cut 1.   Cut 2.   Cut 3.   Cut 4.

Pathway 4 This pathway is the longest (most cuts in a path) of all the paths. You start in at the front, just below pathway 2. Path 4 goes along the upper right side and then back around the upper back part of the head where it meets the back part of paths 1 – 3.

The first 4 or 5 cuts are done while in a 5 o'clock position. As you work your way around the back of the head to the last cut, you change your body's position a little with each cut you make until you are in a 8 or 9 o'clock position.

Assuming an average shaped head, this path goes along one of the major curves of the head. Either your holding fingers conform to this rounded shape, or you'll have to go back and cut an extra path between (overlapping) this path and path 2, **after** you've made the cuts in this path (pages 64 and 65 described this in more detail).

The guide-hair is at the "V" of your holding fingers. It may take as many as 9 – 10 cuts, or as few as 5, to reach the left rear corner.

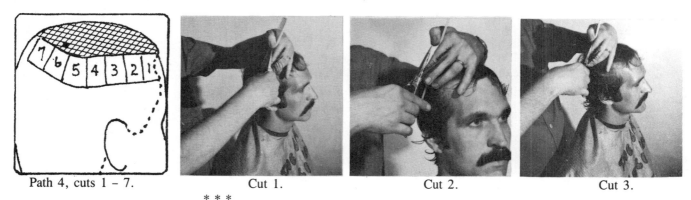

Path 4, cuts 1 – 7.   Cut 1.   Cut 2.   Cut 3.

* * *

Nothing is really work unless you would rather be doing something else.
                                                                James M. Barrie

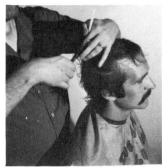
Cut 4.

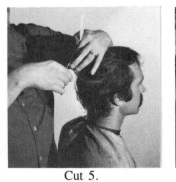
Cut 5.

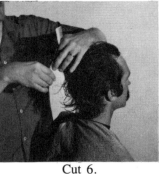
Cut 6.

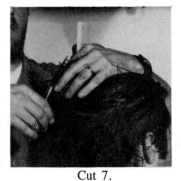
Cut 7.

Don't be afraid of the cowlick back there—stay with your equal-length cutting—it lies fine if the hair is allowed to lie the way it wants.
Pathway 5 For me, the easiest way to handle this pathway is to stand at the 10 – 11 o'clock position and use the comb-away hand-tool manipulation. You can use the basic manipulation at 6 – 7 o'clock, but to me, it feels awkward with my arm up so high. With the basic manipulation the guide-hair is at the fingertips; with the comb-away it shows at the "V" of the holding fingers.

My preferred method using the comb-away requires you to take extra care when positioning your HGH. There is a tendency to have the holding fingertips a bit closer to the scalp than the length at the "V". Just keep this in mind and guard against it. Remember, the comb-away has the points of the blades moving toward the face: go slow and be aware. Path 5 is another curved area—handle it as you did path 4.

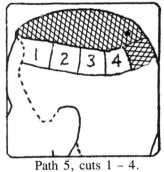
Path 5, cuts 1 – 4.

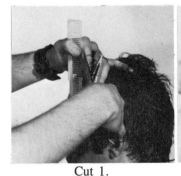
Cut 1.

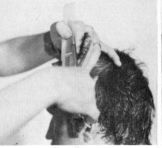
Cut 2.

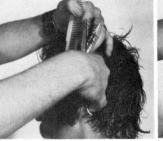
Cut 3.

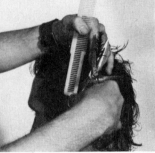
Cut 4.

The alternative approach.

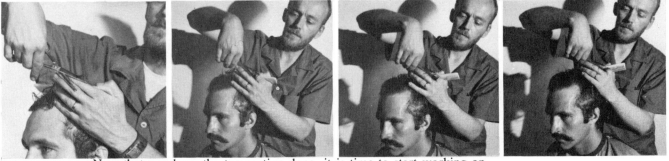

Now that you have the top section done, it is time to start working on the side hair.

B. Right Side Section

For cutting the sides and back sections, have the haircuttee sit on a low chair for the best line of vision. When you cut around the sides and back the guide-hair **always** shows at the "V" of your holding fingers. You will have this guide-hair to use on all the cutting you do, except for:

● Path 1 on the right section—this is another "trail blazer" path like the first one on the top section.

● The first cut in path 3 (right section) behind the right ear; and the first couple of cuts you make in path 1 going up the back section. This area behind the ear, down to the bottom of the back is new territory without neighboring cuts to rely on.

<u>Pathway 1</u> Stand at a 7 to 9 o'clock position with the haircuttee helping by bending his or her neck and head toward you. Always comb the hair straight down on the sides and back before starting out on any of the pathways. Usually you'll make 2 – 3 cuts in this pathway, but make as many cuts as needed to get up to the cut hairs on the top section. As with the first path on the top section, go through this beginning pathway twice to be sure you have it cut evenly.

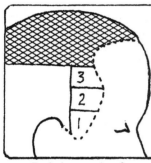
Path 1, cuts 1 – 3.

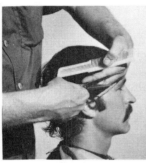
Cut 1.

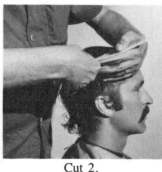
Cut 2.

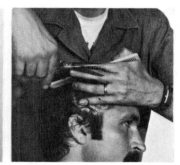
Cut 3.

Because of the irregular shape of the temple's hairline, in some of your manipulations going up this first pathway you will hold and cut small amounts of hair. What you want to do with this first path is get it relatively **straight** so the next couple of paths can also be straight. These in-line pathway routes are much easier to handle than twisted ones that follow the hairline.

<u>Pathway 2</u> Pathway 2 is directly above the ear and you need to take care when starting your comb-out so you don't snag the top of the ear with the comb.

Use the sideways comb trick or the helping-hand method, or you could have the haircuttee fold down the top of their ear. Stay in the 7 – 9 o'clock position.

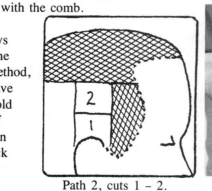
Path 2, cuts 1 – 2.

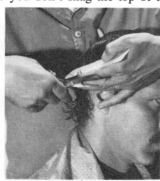
Cut 1.

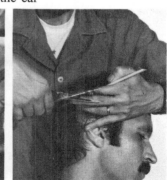
Cut 2.

<u>Pathway 3</u> The last pathway on the right section starts behind the ear, at about mid-ear level. The first cut won't have any guide-hair to use, but the rest of the cuts have it. It might be helpful to have the haircuttee fold their ear forward so it's out of your way. Stand at a 7 – 8 o'clock position.

This pathway may get you into one of the major curve areas of the head. If the head curves, be sure your holding fingers conform, or you could employ the straight approach with the extra pathway between this path and the next one. 4 – 5 cuts will get you up to the top section's cut hair.

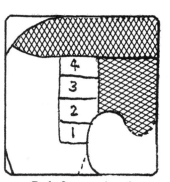

Path 3, cuts 1 – 4.

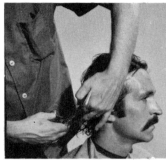

Cut 1.

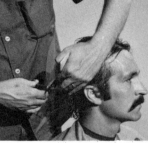

Cut 2.

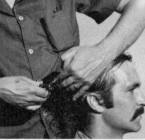

Cut 3.

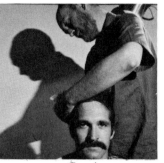

Cut 4.

C. Back Section

When you cut the hair on the lower portion of the back of the head, you can make some changes in the all-the-same-length cutting you have been striving for. Besides an equal-length cutting on the back, you have the following options:

● This area can be tapered in shorter than the rest of the bulk-cutting. If this is what you want, you continue with the equal-length cutting as shown—the 2-step tapering procedure is done after you have finished all the equal-length, bulk-removal. This tapering method is shown on pages 115 through 117 in this chapter.

● The hair can be left longer than the rest of your bulk-cutting. If this longer approach is what you want, skip ahead **now** to page 117 and 118 to see how it's done.

Back to our equal-length cutting. Pathway 1 on the back section is usually on another major curve—do what you have to in order to have your cutting conform to it. You may find it helpful to have the ear folded forward. Stand at the 7 – 8 o'clock position for the first pathway. For each succeeding pathway you move toward the front left side of the haircuttee, until you are at the 10 – 11 o'clock position for the last pathway in this back section.

Pathway 1 As usual, you start by combing the hair down.

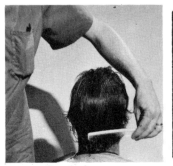

Comb down.

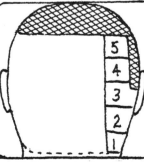

Path 1, cuts 1 – 5.

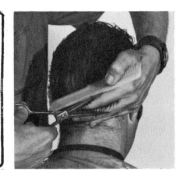

Cut 1.

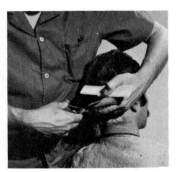

Cut 2.

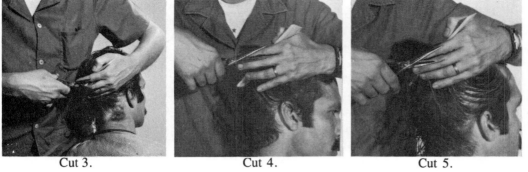

Cut 3.   Cut 4.   Cut 5.

It may take
6 – 7 cuts to
work your way
up to the top
section. One
cut per inch
gets you
there.

The first 2 – 3 cuts in this path are below path 3 on the right side section—you won't have guide-hair to use until about the third cut.

Pathway 2
You will have
guide-hair at
the "V" of the
holding fingers
for all
remaining cuts
in the bulk-
removal.

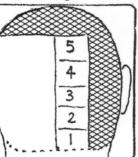

Path 2, cuts 1 – 5.

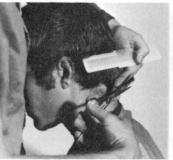

Cut 1.

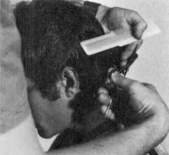
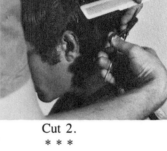

Cut 2.

* * *

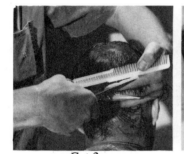

Cut 3.

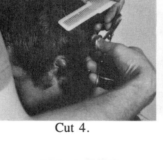

Cut 4.

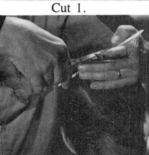

Cut 5.

If you want to
leave your
footprints in the
sands of time,
wear work shoes.
                    Anonymous
Without work all
life goes rotten.
                    Albert Camus

Pathway 3

Path 3, cuts 1 – 5.

Cut 1.

Cut 2.

Cut 3.

* * *

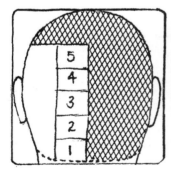

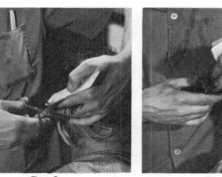

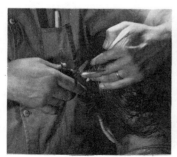

Cut 4.   Cut 5.

You can always tell a real friend:
when you make a fool of yourself he
doesn't feel you've done a
permanent job. Laurence J. Peter
When you're with someone and
silence is comfortable, you are
with a friend.   Anonymous
Please everyone and you please no
one.   Anonymous

Pathway 4 You can do this last back path at the 11 o'clock position or move to 3 – 4 o'clock. Here again, you're working on a major curve area: handle it as you have the previous ones.

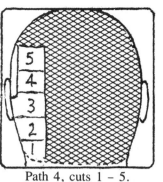

Path 4, cuts 1 – 5.

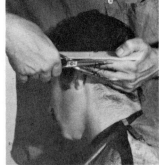

Cut 1.

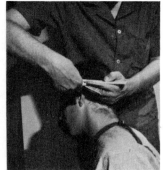

Cut 2.

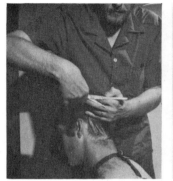

Cut 3.

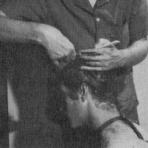

Cut 4.

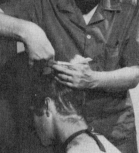

Cut 5.

* * *

Before I judge my neighbor, let me walk a mile in his moccasins.

Sioux proverb

If you judge people you have no time to love them.

Mother Teresa

D. **Left Side Section**

Pathway 1 If you didn't switch over to the right side for the last pathway, get into the 3 – 4 o'clock position for this one. Have the haircuttee fold their ear forward if needed. About 4 cuts will do it.

* * *

When I get to be a psychologist, I'll direct all my patients to go and make something with their hands and give it to someone.   Anonymous

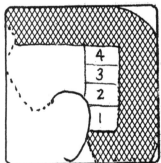

Path 1, cuts 1 – 4.

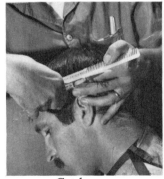

Cut 1.

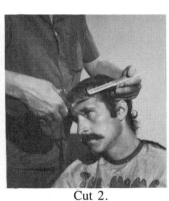

Cut 2.

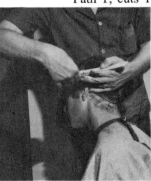

Cut 3.

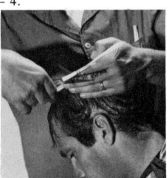

Cut 4.

You could make an extra "pass" through this first pathway to cut off those longer hairs that always seem to be left behind the ear. I recommend that you hold off and take care of it with an extra pathway after you have finished cutting this section. The next page shows how this extra pathway is done.

Pathway 2 Here again, you use whatever means are necessary to start out without snagging the top of the ear with the comb. 2 – 3 cuts gets you to the cut hair on top.

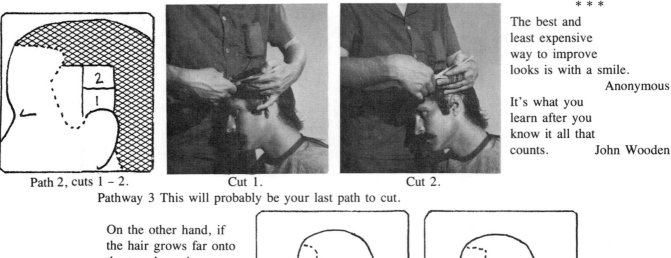

Path 2, cuts 1 – 2.   Cut 1.   Cut 2.

Pathway 3 This will probably be your last path to cut.

On the other hand, if
the hair grows far onto
the temple region, you
may have to make one
extra path to finish
the left side section.

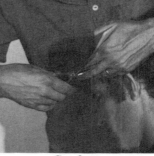

Unusual hairline.   Normal hairline.

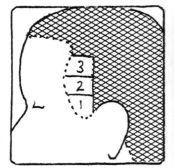 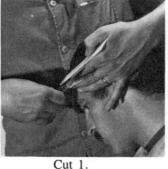 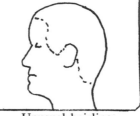 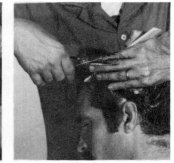

Path 3, cuts 1 – 3.   Cut 1.   Cut 2.   Cut 3.

If the left side needs the extra pathway at the front of this section,
do it now. Before you can consider yourself done with the
bulk-removal, you need to do just a bit more cutting behind the left
ear. For some reason, that area behind the ear doesn't get cut as
evenly as the rest. To remedy this, move to a 11 o'clock position for
this remedial cutting. This may look a little awkward, but I have
found it to be the most effective way to smooth off this area. If
needed, have your haircuttee help by folding the ear forward.

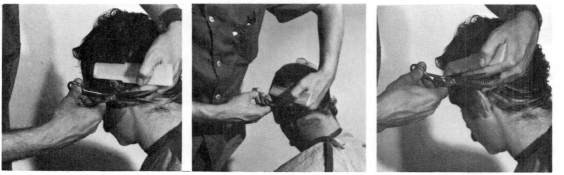

Cut 1.   Cut 2.   Cut 3.

While you're
at it, take
an 8 o'clock
position and
check for
longer hairs
behind the
right ear.

If you aren't going to taper the back-bottom area hair, you have now
finished the first-time-through bulk-removal cutting.

HOORAY FOR HOME HAIRCUTTERS!

8.5 TWO APPROACHES TO CUTTING NECK HAIR

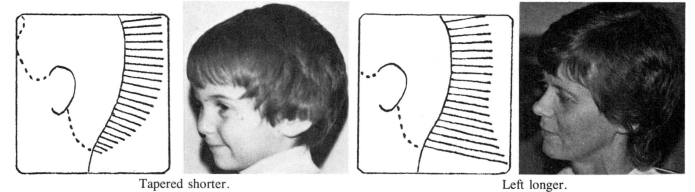

Tapered shorter.   Left longer.

A. 2-Step Tapering

If you are going to taper in the back-bottom hair, making it shorter
than the rest of the hair, now is the time to do it.

For purposes of illustration, let's
say you have given a 3 inch
equal-length cut, with 3 inches of
hair hanging below the neck's
hairline.

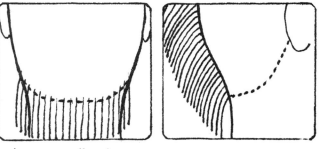

Step 1 Using the finger-bracing-the-scissors or pull-and-cut
method, cut off 1 1/2 – 2 inches of the hair. Leave 1 – 1 1/2 inches
of hair below the hairline. Round the corners a bit.

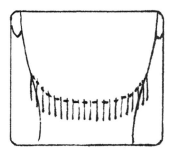 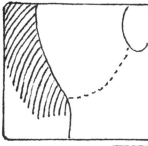 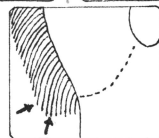

This straight across, blunt
cutting leaves the hair quite
heavy at the cutting line. As
these illustrations show, the
heaviness comes from above,
and that's where step 2 comes
in.

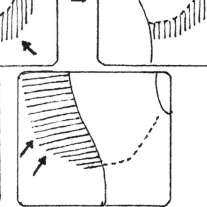

Step 2 If you were to stop after the first step, the hair would
appear as if it had been given a "bowl-cut", and it would tend to be
flippy and shaggy around the bottom.

* * *

All my best thoughts were stolen by the ancients.   Ralph Waldo Emerson
Examine the contents, not the bottle.   The Talmud
There is nothing permanent except change.   Heraclitus
To be wronged is nothing unless you continue to remember it. Confucius
I am a citizen, not of Athens or Greece, but of the world.   Socrates

To get this hair to lie well,
you will concentrate your next
cutting/tapering efforts 1 – 2
inches above the edge hair.
You want the kind of smoothness
shown in the illustration at
the right.

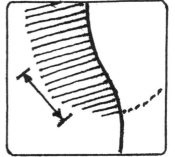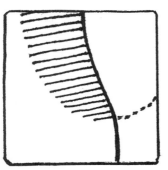

To smooth off this uneven, heavy hair, you will switch to a
diagonal HGH positioning, with your fingertips pointing toward
the neck. This diagonal position has your HGH curve away from the
neck, with your fingertips touching or close to touching the neck.

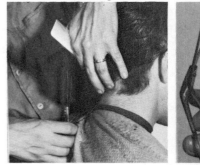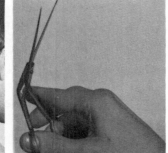

If you were to use a vertical HGH
position with the holding fingers
curved away from the neck, you
would need bent scissors to cut
the held hair—that neck gets in
your way.

Stand at a 7 o'clock position
as you start at the right side.
Have the head bent forward and
down as far as possible. When
you have worked over to the
left side (one cut per inch of
travel), you'll be standing at
a 9 – 10 o'clock position.

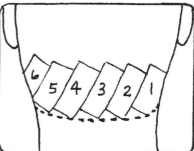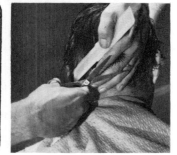

As you can see above, here we begin to cut back on the use of photos;
this will be the case until we get to the edging part of the haircut.

When your HGH is positioned, you want to have
guide-hair showing at the fingertips and the
"V" of the holding fingers. This may require
that you pull your HGH out from the scalp for
some distance. Just cut the longer hair
between the helping hairs to get this hair
smoothed off.

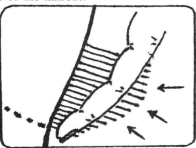

After you have finished this path, make one more path across the back,
just above the previous one to check for smoothness. Here you will be
able to use a vertical position because the neck won't be in your way.
Trim as needed while using guide-hair at the fingertips (from the
previous path) and at the "V" (the already-cut hair above from the
first-time-through cutting).

     If the head of hair you're working on has a fairly strong ducktail
neckline, you may have to use the comb-away method for the bottom,
right side neck hair (see page 121 for more on this.)

     While I recommend this 2-step method of tapering neck hair for the
beginner—it's also used on other tapered cutting you will do—it is

not my preferred method on the neck area. I get the same results, but much quicker, by using a stepping-out method on the first-time-through bulk-removal. With this approach I increase the length I leave the hair with each manipulation made while going up a pathway on the back of the head. Repeating the same stepping-out cuts on each pathway in the back, gets the hair fairly well tapered, ready for a little smoothing off on the second-time-through cutting.

How many stepping-out cuts are made and what length to leave them are questions that depend on the overall length of the rest of the hair, and on what the person likes. This example is fairly typical:

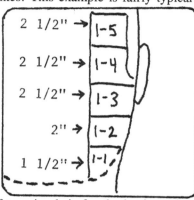

When you give a 2 1/2 inch equal-length cut, the first cut at the neckline leaves the hair 1 1/2 inches long. Move up one inch for the next cut in the pathway and here you leave the hair 2 inches long. Another inch up and you are at the 2 1/2 inch cutting length that is maintained for the rest of the cuts up the pathway.

After you cut this first path, repeat the same length-producing cuts on each of the back's pathways. The guide-hair aid is used after the first path is cut.

I don't recommend this way of tapering hair for the beginner because I feel it requires a level of skill that is too difficult for some. If you think you can do it, go ahead and use it—but you ought to be able to handle this faster way of tapering after you have some experience.

B. Longer Shaping for Neck Hair

To achieve a gradually longer length to the back hairs, comb the hair at the bottom of the neck up, and make the first cut in the pathway **higher up** than you do for equal-length cutting.

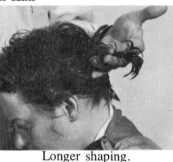
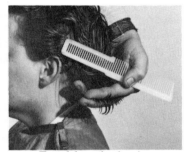

Longer shaping.   Equal-length shaping.

With the hair below the HGH combed up farther—while held at the same length-producing position used on the rest of the bulk-removal cuts—the hair toward the bottom hairline is left gradually longer.

For example, if your HGH is positioned 2 inches up from the hairline, the hair is left with this extra length:

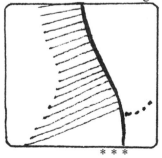

The higher up the first cut is made, the longer the hair is left. If the first cut is 3 inches up, this would result:

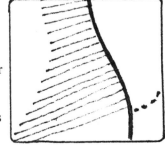

* * *

Use what talent you have—the woods would be very silent if no birds sang except those who sang best.   Anonymous

It is not enough to be busy . . . the question is: what are we busy about?   Henry David Thoreau

The time to relax is when you don't have time to relax.   Anonymous

On the other hand, the lower you make the first cut, the less extra length will be left. If the first cut is 1 inch up from the bottom hairline, this would be the result:

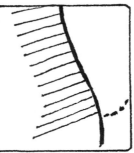

Whatever height you choose, you will repeat it with the first cut on each of the pathways in the back section. The usual starting point is 2 – 2 1/2 inches up for those who like the extra length.

This gradually longer length way to cut can also be done to the bangs. If you had a front hairline cowlick needing a longer length in order to lie well, you comb the hair back and hold it behind the front hairline—the first cut is made there while using the same length-producing position used on the rest of the cuts in the path.

You hold and cut behind the front hairline instead of in the normal, straight-out-from-the-head position, right at the hairline.

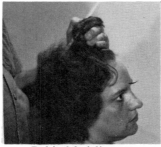

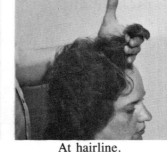

To do this type of shaping, whether it is neck hair or the bangs, the hair at the hairline has to be long enough to reach back, and then up to the holding fingers.

Behind hairline.   At hairline.

NOW TAKE A WELL-EARNED BREAK!

At this point, you have a much deserved rest coming. As a beginner, your arms and hands, even your eyes and brain might be tired. Going ahead if you're pooped might be the worst thing you could do. At this point, the haircut is 80 to 85 percent done, and it won't do any harm if you leave it for a while. Your haircuttee should understand as you take an hour or even a day to recharge your batteries.

8.6 GET IT ALL SMOOTHED OFF

After that deserved rest, you take care of the unevenness that is left from the bulk-cutting. This procedure has two parts to it.

A. Correcting Major Length Differences

Here you are concerned with the hair on one side of the head being left longer than the hair on the other side, or with one side of a section left longer than the other. When you cut hair with the HGH holding the hair, it's very difficult to get an area cut shorter than the rest. However, it is fairly easy for beginners to leave the hair longer, especially by the time you get over to the left side section.

To check the hair's length, pull the hair out in 10 – 12 locations and measure it with a ruler. Differences in length of more than 1/2 inch should be recut as needed.

● If you find a large area of 10 or more square inches, you need to go to an area that is cut to the correct length and check your HGH position there when the hair is held out from the head. Now, go back to the longer area and use the correct HGH position as you recut.

● A small area is done by combing out neighboring, correctly-cut hair and using it as guide-hair while recutting the longer hair.

Rarely (if ever) will you find an area that has been cut too short, but, if you should happen to discover this, you have two options:

(1) Leave it be. For the beginner, I recommend that you accept your boo-boo. Before you give your next haircut, take the time to practice the HGH exercises until you can do them blindfolded.

(2) If the hair can be cut shorter, go back over all the bulk-removal and get the rest of the hair cut as short as your short spot.

If the ruler shows less than 1/2 inch differences in length, they are taken care of with the next part of the smooth off process.

B. Minor Length Differences: The Second-Time-Through Cutting

This "polishing" part of the haircut has just a few photos to show the sequence to use and the position you'll be in. The hair you cut off here may not fill a thimble—that is usually enough to make the difference between a good haircut and an extra good one.

During the second-time-through use the same length-producing position with your HGH as was used on the first-time-through bulk-removal; however, now your HGH is held in a different direction. This change in holding direction reveals the longer than normal culprits that need cutting. As it was with bulk-cutting, you work your way through pathways with the cuts about 1 1/2 – 2 inches wide, and you make one cut for each inch of travel through the path. The main rule for this second cutting is: cut only if needed.

As you go through the entire head of hair, checking for unevenness, many times the hair you hold out from the head doesn't need cutting: good for you—leave it be.

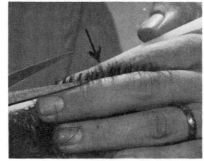

Leave well-enough alone.

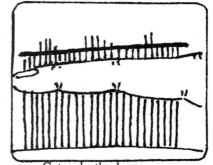

Cut only the longer ones.

I usually ignore unevenness of 1/8 inch or less (the arrow in the photo above points to such a glitch). Yes, this book is about precision haircutting, but if I were to fret about 1/8 inch differences in length, I'd be getting too close to perfectionist haircutting. Whether the uneven hairs you cut are 1/100 or 1/2 inch longer than the rest, be sure that you only cut the longer hairs while using the shorter hairs as a guide—don't cut them.

This part of the haircut needs a systematic sequence of cuts to get all the hair checked over. Doing this with the HGH held in a different direction requires significant changes in how we go about it.

1. **Top Section**. The top hair is divided into 2 halves.

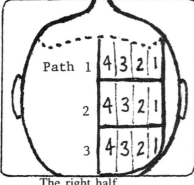

The right half.

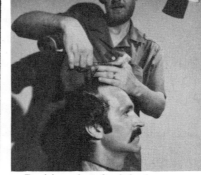

Positioned at 9 o'clock.

On this right section, the holding fingers point toward the crown.

* * *
Forgiveness does not change the past, but it certainly enhances the future.   Anonymous
It's not enough to forgive and forget, we must also forget what we forgave.   Anonymous
A chip on the shoulder indicates there is wood higher up.   Anonymous

The holding fingers point toward the front on this left section.

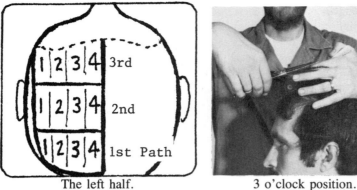

The left half.   3 o'clock position.

Always comb
the hair
away from
you before
making your
cuts through
the pathway.

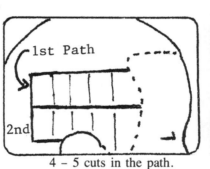

Use the same high stool
for this cutting as was
used for bulk-cutting on
the top section. Keep
using this stool for all
the remaining second-
time-through cutting.

2. Right Side Section.

Here the holding
fingers point to the
bottom hairline. This
is the way it will be
for all the remaining
second-time-through
cutting.

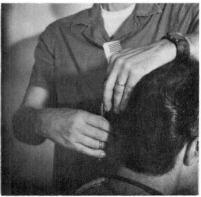

4 – 5 cuts in the path.   5 o'clock position.

The sequence of cuts is not shown in the diagram above because the
sequence you use depends on the grain of the hair. If you're working
on a Type 1 hairgrain, comb the hair to the front, then make 4 – 5
cuts from the front to the back of this section. If the hair has a
Type 2 hairgrain, comb the hair toward the back of the head. Begin at
the back of the section as you use the comb-away method to work your
way forward to the front hairline.

3. Back Section.

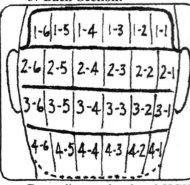

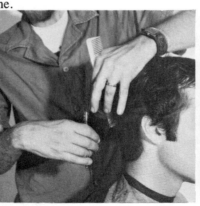

Depending on head and HGH size, you may have as few as 3 paths, or as
many as 5. Position yourself at about 7 o'clock and then move to 9 -
10 o'clock as you get to the end of each pathway. Return to 7 o'clock
for the next, lower pathway.

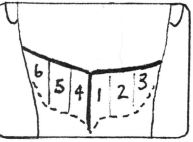

If the hair has a strong ducktail neckline hairgrain, the bottom 1 – 2 paths need the comb-away manipulation on the right side of the neck. Start at the center of the tail and cut toward the right side of the neck; back to the tail, then over to the left side using the basic manipulation.

Note, if you tapered in the bottom neck hair shorter by using the beginner's 2-step method, you already did your second-time-through cutting on the lower pathways. (If you went with the stepping-out method, the hair needs a second-time-through cutting now—use the diagonal HGH positioning for the bottom path.) If you modified your equal-length cutting so as to leave the hair longer at the bottom of the neck, there is **no way** to do this smooth-off cutting with the HGH held in a vertical direction. The only good way to deal with this gradually increasing length is to repeat the same cutting procedure you used to get the increasing length during the first-time-through. As with all your second-time-through cutting, you may not have to shorten a single hair, but checking assures you that it's cut right.

4. **Left Side Section.**

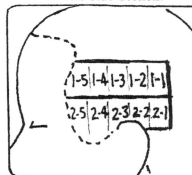
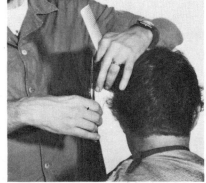
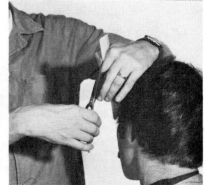

In this last section, you cut 2 paths as you did on the right side. Start out in a 9 – 10 o'clock position and move to 11 o'clock as you get to the end of the pathways. You could reverse the sequence of cuts and use the comb-away method if the hair has a Type 1 grain, but the sequence shown normally works well with Type 1 and Type 2 hairgrains when the basic hand-tool manipulation is used.

This is about the time I get feelings of accomplishment—the hair is shaped-up, and there is just a little more to do. Take a break for a spell and you will be ready for the edges.

8.7 EDGE—CUTTING

This part of the haircut process is similar to the second-time-through cutting in that very little hair needs to be cut. With the exception of the edging you do to the hair covering the ears and possibly the lower temple area hair, all you do is cut off as little as possible.

The sequence of cuts used here makes it possible to rely on guide-hair for nearly all of the cuts (exceptions are pointed out). The idea is to use a bit of the already-cut, neighboring hair as a guide for the next cut you make, whenever possible.

Keep in mind that you want your edgeline cutting to conform to and be equal distance from the hairline. While there are some exceptions to this rule that will be explained with the step-by-step photos, even the exceptions require you to be aware of the shape of the hairline. To be aware, comb the hair back or up and away from its lying position so you can **see** what you have to work with. When you comb the hair back to the cutting position, keep a mental picture of the hairline to which your cutting conforms.

A. **Bangs**. Start on the left side of the bangs while standing at a 3 – 4 o'clock position. Make 3 – 4 cuts using the modified-bulk-removal edging method to get over to the haircuttee's right side.

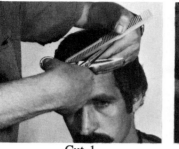 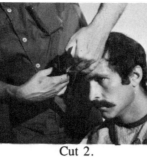 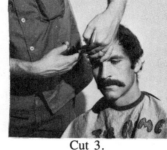

Cut 1.   Cut 2.   Cut 3.

After you've made your first cut, be sure to comb up a little of the cut hair to use as guide-hair for each new cut you make.

Note that due to the 2 inch length the hair was left during the bulk-removal, the HGH has a fanned out position. If it had been left longer (2 1/2 or more inches), the space fingers would be tucked up under the held hair. The pull-and-cut method is a good alternative to this method: this approach requires 11, 12, and 1 o'clock positions.

After you have finished this cutting, move to a 1 o'clock position and comb the hair forward onto the forehead. Use the finger-bracing-the-scissors method to cut any stragglers.

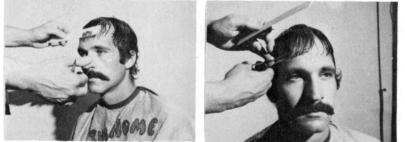

Be sure you don't cut any of the temple region hair when cutting the bangs. Comb the side hair toward the back of the head, so it's out of your way.

It's usually best if the bottom of the bangs are cut so they are equal distance from the front hairline, even if the bangs are to be worn so they lie off to one side. This way of cutting insures the bangs stay in good shape no matter which way they end up lying.

For bangs cutting, the haircuttee sits on a low chair. For the next part of the edging, a high chair is best.

B. **Temple Region—Right Side**.

For our purposes, this part of the edging is divided into two parts. While the hairline in this region can take a variety of shapes, what you see here is fairly typical.

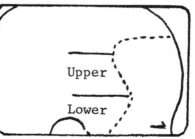

1. **Upper part**. If the head of hair I'm cutting has the common hairline shape shown above and if the hair is straight or wavy, I won't do any edging on the upper part—the hair always lies down (Type

* * *

This country will not be a good place for any of us to live in unless we make it a good place for all of us to live in.   Theodore Roosevelt

1 hairgrain) or toward the back of the head (Type 2 hairgrain), so with no hair lying out on the edges, I just leave it be.

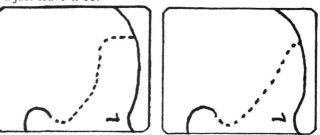

I do the edging on the upper part **only** if I'm working on curlier hair, or if the hair has one of these less common hairlines in the temple region and a Type 1 hairgrain.

This upper temple area is easily cut by using the pull-and-cut method with you in a 12 – 1 o'clock position. As with the bangs, your cutting here will be minimal—just a little trimming does it. Avoid cutting the bangs by combing them toward the haircuttee's left before you begin.

2. **Lower part**. The lower portion, unlike the upper part, always needs a little edging and sometimes, as in the following example, more than just a little. If you've given a longer version of the equal-length cut, most folks, especially those with the straighter hair, need to have this hair cut short enough so it won't end up in the eyes if windblown. Curlier hair usually isn't affected by this problem because of its springy growth: a minimum cutting works well on curls.

If the hair is long enough, you could use the pull-and-cut method, standing at the 1 – 2 o'clock position. A couple of cuts ought to take care of it. (Note my method of cutting: be sure your cutting is done on the inside of the holding fingers, not above them as shown.)

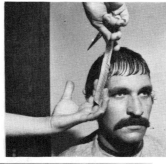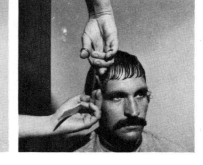

With shorter hair, the finger-bracing method works well, but if the hair wants to lie toward the back of the head, the scissors-and-comb method is needed.

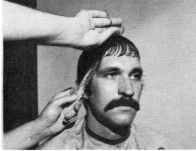

Whatever method you use and however much hair you cut off, you always want the cutting line to be parallel to (equal distance from) the lower temple's hairline.

C. **Right Sideburn**. If your haircuttee doesn't have sideburns, you can skip ahead to the next edging step. Before you start, you need to get the longer side hair above the burns out of the way. You can comb through the side hair as shown here—this gets the hair tucked-in behind the ear.

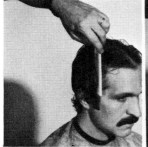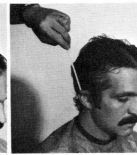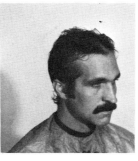

If the hair is too short to be tucked away, you will need a helping hand:

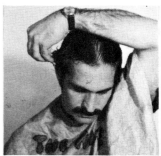

Comb the sideburn hair toward the ear. Use the finger-bracing-the-scissors method to cut the hair close to the sideburn's back hairline. Then comb the hair toward the face and cut on the front hairline:

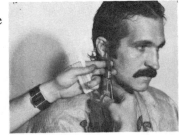 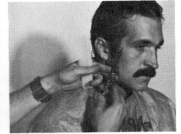

You may have to use the scissors-and-comb method on the frontside or backside cutting, especially with curlier hair. Here you perform this edging method in a little different manner.

Instead of having the comb nearly flat to the skin as you did on the lower temple region, now the comb is held perpendicular to the skin.

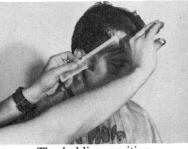

The holding position for the lower temple region.

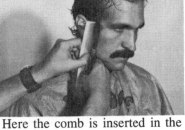

Here the comb is inserted in the middle of the burns and moved to the edge of the front hairline.

Using the scissors-and-comb on the backside of the burns needs this position for the comb. This upside-down approach has to be done with the teeth at the end of the comb. Hold the rest of the comb away from the scalp so you avoid combing into the hair above the burns.

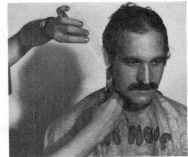 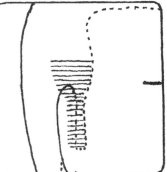

Either way of trimming sideburns works well for straight or wavy hair. However, it may leave curlier hair with the burns too bushy. If this is the case, skip ahead to beard trimming in the last chapter—the scissors-over-comb method shown there will whittle down those burns.

After the sideburns are trimmed, the length of the sideburn hair will be as short as 1/4 inch (scissor-over-comb cutting) to as long as 1/2 inch or a little more (finger-bracing cutting on the sideburn's edges). If the bulk-removal length on the side hair is 1 1/2 inches long or longer, a length difference will exist where the sideburn meets the side hair.

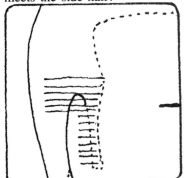

If the side hair is shorter than 1 1/2 inches (so only a little of the ear is covered), those longer side hairs get tapered and blend with the shorter sideburn hair when the edging is done to the side hair. If it needs more tapering, it's done when you do the finishing touches (see page 129).

If you need to raise the bottom of the sideburns, just comb the hair down and use the finger-bracing method with short snips. Move forward 1/8 – 1/4 inch after you make a cut and reopen the scissor blades. This cut-open-move approach leaves a line across the burns that makes it easy to shave the hair left below the line.

How long to leave sideburns is a question without an easy answer. Whatever the person prefers is the obvious choice. For myself, I like to see some sideburn showing beneath the side hair. I also think long burns fit a longer shaped face; shorter burns go with a shorter face.

Trimming sideburns and the rest of the edging around the sides and back, requires a position that has your eyes on the same level as the cutting you do.

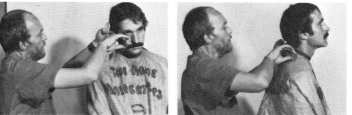

D. **Right Side Hair**. You cut straight across here, ignoring the shape of the hairline. How much hair you leave covering the ear was dealt with back in chapter 6, sections 4 and 5.

First, comb the hair above the ear and in front of the ear forward like this:

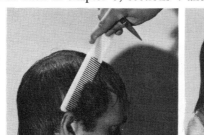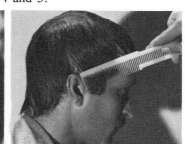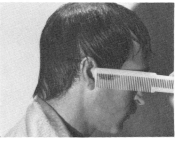

This gets the hair that tends to lie toward the back of the head (above the ears) cut off in front of the ears. They won't appear in front of the ear later, making that part of the edgeline unevenly cut.

Then, comb all the side hair, from the temple hairline to the back of the ear, straight down. Use the pull-and-cut method with the cutting done on the inside of holding hand. Start at the face side and work your way to the back edge of the ear; this takes about 2 – 3 manipulations.

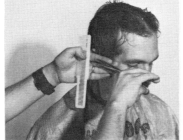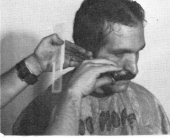

After you cut your straight line to the back edge of the ear, go back to the corner where the lower temple region edging meets the side edging. Round off the corner a little. You can use the pull-and-cut if the hair is long enough, or the scissors-and-comb method I prefer.

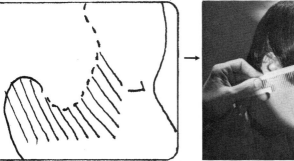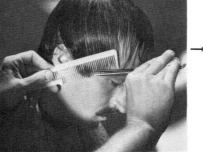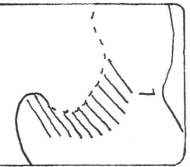

E. **Right Side of the Neck**. Before we begin this edging, you need to know how the different approaches to cutting the lower neck hair (during the bulk-removal) affects the edging line you cut here.

(1) If you gave an equal-length cutting, your edging line follows this kind of path.

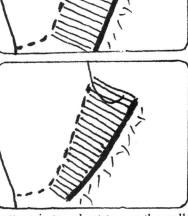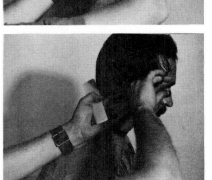

(2) If you tapered in the back bottom hair, the edge-cutting takes this kind of shape.

If the hair toward the bottom is too short to use the pull-anc-cut, use the finger-bracing or scissors-and-comb methods on the shorter portion.

(3) The long cutting approach dictates this kind of edge-cutting line.

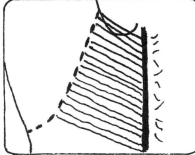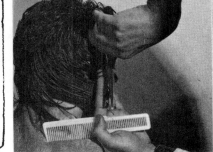

Note that in each case, the hair is pulled straight away from the hairline, and the cutting occurs as close to the skin as possible. With this part of the edging, you return to a minimum cutting.

When cutting the side of the neck edgeline, start where your covering the ear cuts left off. Use that cut hair at the back edge of the ear as guide-hair for your first pull-and-cut. The guide-hair appears (with careful combing) at your finger tips. It takes 2 – 3 pull-and-cuts to get down to the bottom.

F. **Bottom Neckline.** Here you want to cut the edgeline straight across and round the corners (where the bottom meets the sides). The edging method to use depends on how you shaped the lower neck hair during the bulk-removal.

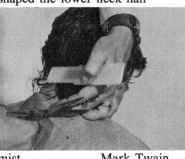

(1) If you gave a long cutting, use the modified-bulk-removal or the pull-and-cut. Going from right to left will take 3 – 4 manipulations with either method.

* * *

There is no sadder sight than a young pessimist.   Mark Twain
Mankind owes to the child the best it has to give.   U.N. Declaration
Today I heard a child laugh—my day is complete.   Anonymous.

(2) Equal-length cutting in the back lends itself to the pull-and-cut, followed by the finger-bracing approach for left-over stragglers.

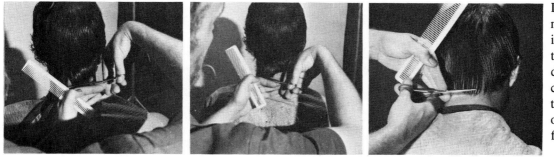

Don't follow my example in the first two photos— do your cutting on the inside of the holding fingers.

(3) The shorter, tapered bulk-cutting usually leaves the bottom hair too short for the pull-and-cut, so use the finger-bracing-the-scissors or the scissors-and-comb method. Start at the right corner and proceed to the left. If you're working on a ducktail neckline, start at the tail and work your way to the right edge—back to the tail and then to the left side.

After you have snipped your way to the left corner, go to the right corner, and round off the area where the two straight edgelines meet.

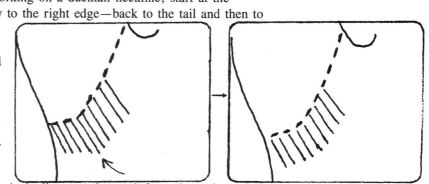

If your haircuttee has a ducktail, remember to inform them about the nature of this hairgrain condition, and that your straight-across cutting line never stays that way. As soon as they bend their neck back or their collar brushes against that straight edgeline, to some extent, it always goes back to its ducktail druthers. Those with this kind of neck hair have had years to adjust to a neckline that has a "mind of its own", so there won't be major disappointment when you prove you're not a magician.

Up to this point, the edging has been done in a fairly consistent sequence of cuts around the head. If you were to go ahead with the left side of the neck's edging now, you would find it difficult to finish this edging at the **right** place on the back edge of the ear. So we jump ahead a little.

G. **Left Sideburn**. If you trimmed the right sideburn, you have a little snipping to do on the left. Do it the same way as the right side, except that here, if you use the scissor-and-comb method, do your upside-down comb handling on the front side of the burns.

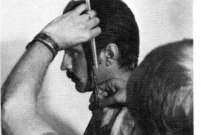

Whatever methods are used, trim it on both sides.

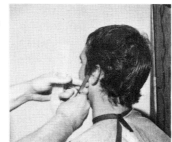

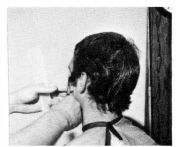

H. **Left Side Hair**. Before you start, comb the hair above the ear in a forward and down direction, as you did it on the right side. Then

go back to the right side and comb that hair down into a pull-and-cut
holding position so you can see exactly where the edgeline was cut
there in relation to the ear. Return to the left and repeat the same
edging line on this side.

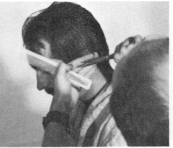

Do this cutting the same way
you did it on the right side,
but here, the first pull-and-
cut is done to the hair that
comes down over the ear. Work
from there, cut by cut,
toward the face.

I. **Left side neck**. This part of the edge-cutting can now be done
with greater assurance that the edgeline will start off and end up
where you want it.

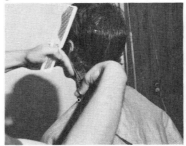

On the first pull-and-cut,
use the cut hair that covers
the ear as guide-hair (on
this side, the guide-hair is
at the "V" of the holding
fingers). Remember to do the
pull-and-cut on the inside
of the holding fingers.
Be sure to keep in mind and duplicate the edgeline you cut on the
right side of the neck. After you've reached the bottom, round off the
corner as you did on the right side.

J. **Left side temple hair**.
For this last part of the
edging, stand in a 10 – 11
o'clock position. Do the
cutting the same way you
did on the right side—the
difference here is your
cutting goes from the
bottom toward the top.

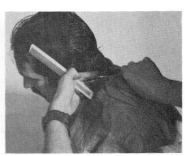

Lower temple.   Upper temple if needed.

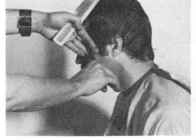

The last of the edging is the corner where
the lower temple and side hair meet. On
this side I use the finger-bracing method
after the side hair has been combed toward
the corner. You can also use the pull-and-
cut or the scissors-and-comb method.

You're done with the edging—**THREE CHEERS FOR DO-IT-YOURSELFERS!**
After you've given yourself a few pats on the back, it's on to the
finishing touches.

8.8 FINISHING TOUCHES

The finishing touches are to a haircut like gift wrapping is to a nice
gift. We begin with last minute hair concerns for the fellows.
● Post-adolescent males may need extra hairgrowth trimmed at the

eyebrows, ears, and nose (see chapter 6, section 14 for the how-to).
● Extra hairs at the bottom and sides of the neck can be cut shorter in several ways (page 91 described a couple of methods). Here I sue close-cutting clippers to remove those extra hairs. The clipper is positioned as shown, then it moves downward.

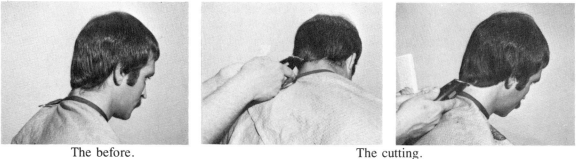

The before.   The cutting.

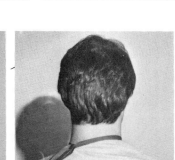

The same results are achieved by using soap lather and a safety razor. Start shaving where the scissors' cutting left off.

The finished product.

A growing number of fellows prefer the same scissors-over-comb cutting that women usually have done to their extra neck hairs. This approach, like eyebrow trimming, leaves the hair fairly short, but not with a freshly-cut appearance.

● Trimming the beard. When you give a haircut to a gent with a beard, you usually find that the beard no longer fits the new haircut. It is time to do some more trimming—the last chapter goes into detail.

    Now we do those finishing touches that apply to all your haircuts.

1. **Longer Hairs in Front of the Ears**. Use the combing technique shown for the right side hair (page 125) to be sure there are no longer hairs around the ear area.

2. **Back of the Ear Surplus**. Try as I may, I almost always end up with a chunk of longer hairs where the covering-the-ear edgeline meets the side-of-the-neck edgeline. To take care of that, I use what I call the pinch-pull-cut method.

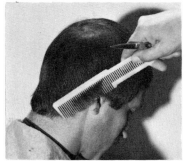
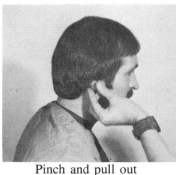
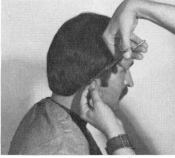

This method can be used anywhere around the edges where longer hairs show up.

Comb through the hair.   Pinch and pull out the longer hairs.   Cut as close to the finger and thumb as possible.

3. **Tapering the Hair that Covers the Ear**. If you cut off 3/4 inch or more during the edging on the hair that covers the ear, that hair will be in the same condition neck hair is in after doing the first step in the 2-step tapering method. To remove this flippy-prone hair,

use the same diagonal cutting approach you used during the second part of the tapering. Just a little tapering done to the longer hairs from above will leave the hair lying smoothly.

4. **The Final Eyeballing**. After you have drummed the hair dry, comb or brush the hair into its preferred lying position. Look in a mirror or step back a couple of yards. Check for a sloping neckline, uneven bangs, or unevenness anywhere it may show itself. Also look for any heaviness or cutting lines that might be left from the bulk-removal. As chapter 6, section 13 pointed out, when making corrections on straighter hair, you comb out the hair above (on the sides and back sections) and behind (on the top section), from where you see the unevenness. Remember, the general rule to follow with flippy hair is to cut it a little shorter: the exception occurs with coarse, straight hair and a ducktail neckline—here you leave the hair extra long or it must be cut extra short.

5. **The Fun Part**. With the hair combed or brushed so those ends are like carefully positioned shingles, show the haircuttee a mirror. (A hand mirror used with a wall mirror allows them to see the back of the head.) Take the time to show them what a healthful scalp massage is, followed by a handcombing. Give them the mirror again—the contrast between the hair before cutting, and what they see now, will convince them that a precision haircut makes **all** the difference.

6. **Healthy Haircare**. Share what you know about hair damage and how easy it is to make hair as healthy as can be. Keep in mind that if the hair has been damaged by chemicals, heat appliances, thinning shears, or from razor cutting, the hair will probably need 1 – 2 more haircuts before the damaged hair is grown out enough to be all cut off. During this time, the haircuttee **must** change their damaging ways if they are to correct their condition. Healthy haircare is simple, but it needs to be practiced **everyday**.

There you have it, the world's most commonly given haircut. I strongly recommend that you stay with it until you're thoroughly comfortable with the haircutting process. After you have worked off your rough edges on this versatile haircut, you will be ready for the two more difficult haircuts. You will advance, but you will come back to this cut again and again—this basic cut will always be in demand.

* * *

No one is useless in this world who lightens the burdens of another.
                                                              Charles Dickens
There is no higher religion than human service. To work for the common good is the greatest creed.   Albert Schweitzer
It's what we value—not what we have—that makes us rich.
                                                              Dr. J. Harold Smith
Those who need help are not near as needy as those who refuse to give it.   Anonymous
Selfishness is at the root of virtually every hurtful, evil-minded act ever commited.   Bob Ohnstad
Repay evil with good and you deprive the evildoer of all the pleasures of his wickedness.   Leo Tolstoy
There is nothing noble in being superior to other men, true nobility is being superior to your former self.   Anonymous
I am not the man I ought to be, nor am I the man I want to be, but thank God I am not the man I used to be.   Alcoholics Anonymous saying
Plant your own garden and decorate your own soul, instead of waiting for someone to bring you flowers.   Anonymous

9.1 INTRODUCTION

This chapter teaches the best (to my way of thinking) and most skilled way of giving a long haircut. First you will learn the most common version of a long, layered cut along with the new ways of using your hands and tools. Then you'll learn some of the different ways this basic haircut can be shaped. Concentrate your beginner's efforts on the first shaping, and with that experience in your bag of skills, you'll be able to handle the variations on this haircut.

     The first sets of photos reveal the transformation this haircut brings to a head of hair. The last row of photos on the next page show only the finished product (while busy working at the haircut shop, sometimes the before photo doesn't come to mind until after the cutting is done).

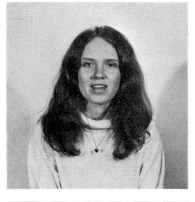

Flat line shape
with top, center
path cut to 3
inch length.

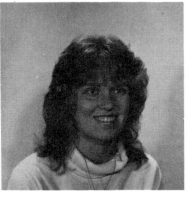

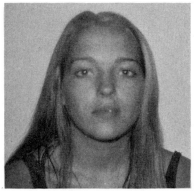

Type 2, straight, fine
to medium texture.
Cowlick on front
hairline and troublesome
ducktail. Same cutting
as one on left.

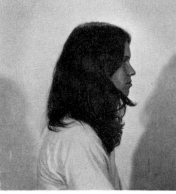

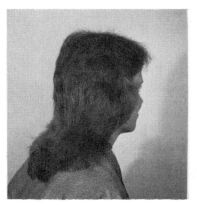

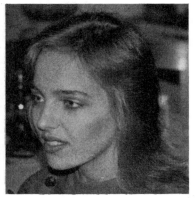

Cross between Type 1
and 2, slightly wavy,
medium texture. Has
only had perimeter
trims in past 5 years.

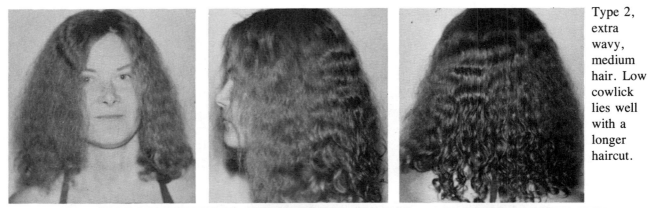

Type 2, extra wavy, medium hair. Low cowlick lies well with a longer haircut.

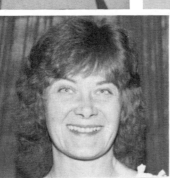

Cut to 3 inch length length on top, center path. Flat line shape.

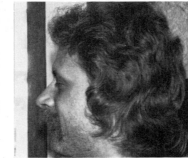

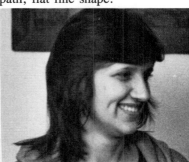

Type 2, straight, medium hair. 2 1/2 inches on top 3 paths. Umbrella shape.

Type 1, wavy, medium hair. 2 inches on top, center path. Flat line shape.

Type 1, straight, medium to coarse hair. 3 1/2 inch top, center path, flat line shape.

The end of chapter 2 described how there are two basic ways to cut long hair. The easy way for the haircutter is the perimeter trim: the hair is combed down and snipped off on the bottom edges. A long, layered cut isn't as easy to cut, but it's much easier to care for on a daily basis. The easy haircut leaves a lot of hair on the head.

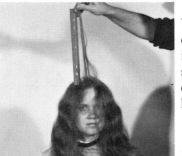

With the long, layered cut, over half of this top hair is cut off, but the way it's shaped and the precision cutting makes the hair look long.

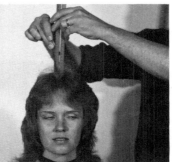

Chapter 2 also explained the advantages of the long, layered cut. While this haircut can't be braided or put into a ponytail as can the perimeter haircut, its lack of tangles and snarls and other easy care features makes it, like the equal-length cut, another people-pleaser.

9.2 SOME CHANGES FROM THE EQUAL-LENGTH HAIRCUT

With the equal-length cut, all the holding-guide-hand (HGH) had to do was lock into the same length-producing position while conforming to the shape of the head throughout the bulk-removal. With this long cut, your HGH still operates as a spacer tool while holding the hair away from the head, but there are some differences.

● The bottom of the HGH won't always have the head to rest on.

● On some parts of the haircut, the hair is held out from the head in a different direction.

● The sequence of cuts is similar to that used on the equal-length cut, but there are also significant changes.

● The edging on this cut does not depend on the shape of the hairline; here the edging conforms to the overall shape of the bulk-cutting.

9.3 THE CUTTING LINE

With a long, layered cut, the shortest hair is on top of the head—the farther down you go on the sides or back, the longer the hair gets:

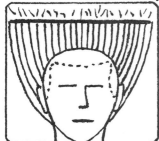 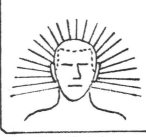 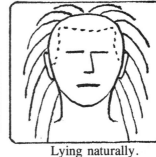 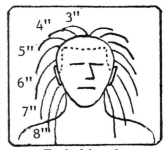

| Cutting line. | Electrified shape. | Lying naturally. | Typical lengths. |

This haircut would be extra easy if the haircuttee could be hung upside-down during your cutting.

All you would have to do is brush the hair down and let gravity keep it that way. Then merely cut it straight across as if you were cutting an upside-down hedge.

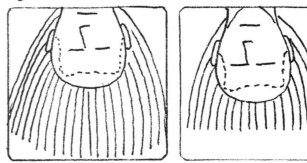

Without the convenience of this haircutting position, your haircutting efforts become a bit more difficult, but still very achieveable. On your first long, layered cut, you will go after the same **flat** cutting line shown on the upside-down model. However, you'll handle the hair in some new ways to make this flat cutting line happen with a person in the upright position.

9.4 CUT-BY-CUT BULK-REMOVAL

A. Preliminary Cutting
Removing hard-to-handle hair is easy with this technique.

* * *

If one advances confidently in the direction of his dreams, and endeavors to live the life which he has imagined, he will meet with a success unexpected in common hours.   Henry David Thoreau

All you do is brush all of the hair up to the top center of the head as if you were going to make a pony-tail. Then cut all the hair above the hand.

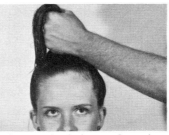 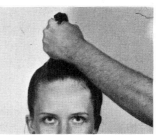

This one-snip approximate cutting leaves the hair **much** easier to handle. Do this whenever you have 3 or more inches of hair to cut off. Preliminary edging isn't necessary when you give the one-snip cut, but if you want, go to the section on edging and follow along. Leave the hair several inches longer than the desired final length on the edges.

B. Cutting the Top

These are the same first 3 paths, with the same sequence of cuts in the paths, that was used on the equal-length cut.

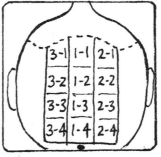

<u>Pathway 1</u> Hold your HGH straight up from the scalp, and rest the bottom of the hand on the scalp. This leaves the hair about 3 inches long—a length that nearly always works well (if a shorter length is desired, read section 6-A now). Due to the flat cutting line, your holding fingers are held straight across rather than conforming to to the shape of the head (as they did with the equal-length cut).

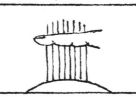 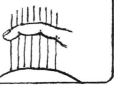

Stand at a 6 o'clock position and comb the top hair forward. The first photo shows how to make the hair easier to handle for the first comb up and cut.

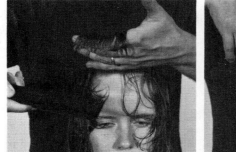

Helping-hand aid.

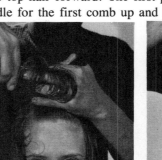

Cut 1.

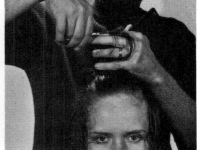

Cut 2.

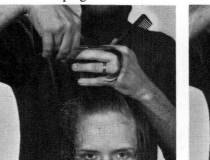

Cut 3.

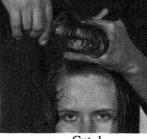

Cut 4.

After you make your cuts, recomb the hair toward the front and cut this path a second time. Comb the hair forward again, and you're ready for the second path.

<u>Pathway 2</u>Depending on how flat or oval the top of the head is, you may only have the wrist resting on the head while cutting this path. In any case, continue the flat cutting line you established with the first pathway's cutting. To that end you have two important aids:
(1) Be sure the comb up includes some of the first pathway's already-cut hair. That helpful guide-hair in your holding hand's grasp shows you how much to cut off.
(2) Keep a clear mental picture of the flat cutting line you are after, with your holding fingers held just below that line.

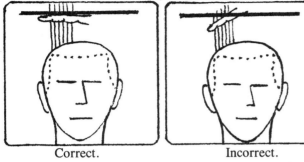

Correct.   Incorrect.

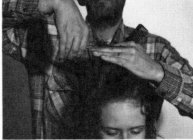

Some prefer this HGH position.

For myself, the more relaxed HGH position shown in the cut-by-cut photos works best.

To help you keep this cutting line in mind, do the top cutting with the haircuttee sitting on a high chair. (I would have liked to have the haircuttee sitting 3 – 4 inches higher, but the chair used at the photographer's studio didn't allow this.) This lower chair may be less arm-tiring, but when you look down on the top, it's much easier to get away from the flat cutting line we are after.

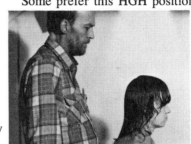

As this first photo shows, you can stand at a 1 o'clock position and use the comb-away method. My preference shows after the first cut.

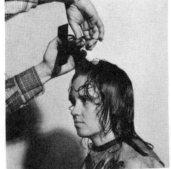

Cut 1.

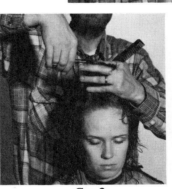

Cut 2.

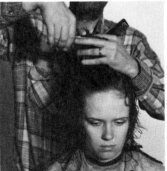

Cut 3.

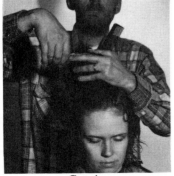

Cut 4.

The arrow points to guide-hair at the "V" of the holding fingers when standing at 6 o'clock. If you're at 1 o'clock using the comb-away method, the guide-hair is at the finger tips.

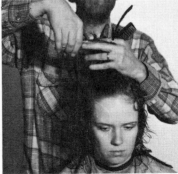

Guide hair at the "V".

<u>Pathway 3</u> This last top pathway, like the second, can be done from either a front or back position. I prefer to position myself in front of the haircuttee at about 11 o'clock, and use the comb-away method. Use either the front or back position—whatever you're comfortable

with. If you stand in front, the guide-hair appears at the "V".

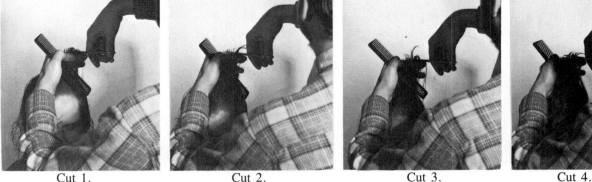

Cut 1.   Cut 2.   Cut 3.   Cut 4.

Before we move on to the next part, go back and repeat each of the
cuts in pathways 2 and 3. The idea is to be sure this first part of
the haircut is done as well as possible because that top hair is much
used as guide-hair for the cutting you do next.

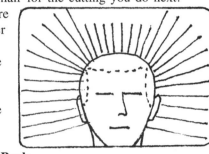

If the hair were
electrified after
the top three
pathways have
been cut, it
would appear
something like
this:

The next part of the haircut
removes this unevenness. At
the same time, the hair
around the sides and back
will be evenly-cut with a
gradually increasing length
to it.

C. Sides and Back

In the equal-length haircut you followed a next-door-neighbor sequence
of paths around the sides and back of the head, and each pathway had
2 – 6 cuts as you moved up the path. With the long, layered cut you
follow the same sequence of pathways, but instead of 2 – 6 cuts, you
comb up **all** of the hair in the pathway—up to the already-cut top
hair—and cut it off with just one snip.

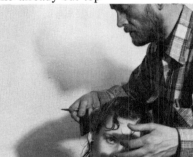

For your best vision and tool handling ease,
seat your haircuttee on a low chair and
stand at 9 o'clock. With some head bending
help, you'll have the line of vision shown
here.

This is how you go about it:

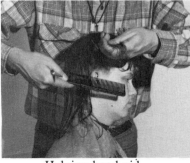

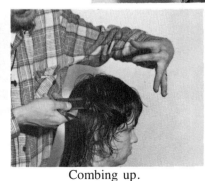

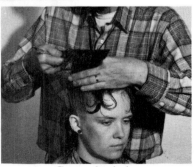

Helping hand aid.   Combing up.   Grasp the hair.

* * *

My riches consist not in the extent of my possessions, but in the
fewness of my wants.
                                                           J. Brotherton

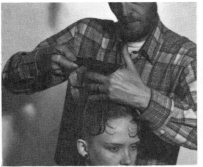

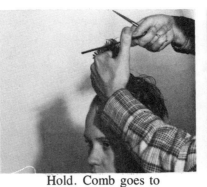

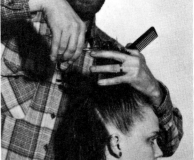

Slide the HGH up to cutting position.

Hold. Comb goes to the resting place.

The cut.

1. **How Much to Cut Off?** To cut off the right amount of side and back hair, you must comb up into the cut hair on the outside edge of the top section: this allows you to include some of the already-cut top hair (guide-hair) in your HGH's grasp. That guide-hair is easily seen by you if you stand on the side opposite that part of the head you're working on. For example, if you're cutting the right side hair, you stand to the haircuttee's left; when you work on the back, you stand in front.

With the equal-length cut, your guide-hair always appeared at the "V" or the finger tips.

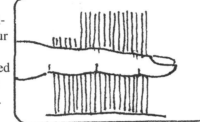

Now it shows up as short hairs against a background of longer hairs.

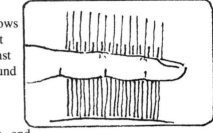

You need careful combing to get the guide-hair into your grasp, and you need to look closely to see it. Cut off **all** the longer hairs that protrude above the shorter guide-hair. Take care not to cut any of those helpful hairs.

2. **Positioning the HGH**. Once you have the long side hair and the short top hair in your HGH, slide your spacer tool (with a pinching pressure between the holding fingers) **straight up** until you have 1/8 – 1/4 inch of guide-hair protruding above the holding fingers—

stop right there. At this point your holding fingers are just beneath and parallel to the flat cutting line. You can use the more relaxed positioning for the HGH, or the flat hand approach.

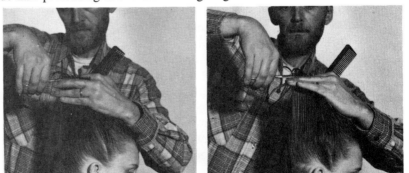

3. **Comb Handling**. You will deal with some long, cumbersome hair when you comb up the pathways around the sides and back. The preliminary cutting minimizes this, and to make it easier when you begin the comb up, make good use of the helping-hand aid and the sideways method of starting out. There are a few more things to know about the comb handling you'll do.

● Uncovering the guide-hair. After you comb up the sides or back hair and slide your HGH up to the cutting position, you may find the

* * *

Honesty is the first chapter of the book of wisdom.   Thomas Jefferson

longer, uncut hair curves over and covers the guide-hair when the comb
is transfered to its resting place. The remedy is easy: comb the long
hairs away from you and the covered-up guide-hair is exposed. Now the
comb goes to its resting place and you can proceed with cutting.

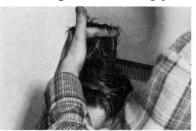
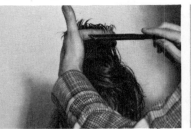
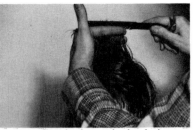

| The guide-hair is covered up. | Flip your wrist so the teeth of the comb are pointed away from you. | Comb through the hair so the guide-hair is exposed. |

● The hairs that don't reach up to the cutting. You may find that some
of the lower hair (the hair toward the bottom of the pathway you comb
up) is not long enough to reach all the way up to the top area where
you cut.

Don't worry about those
hairs. All you have to be
concerned with is the hair
that's long enough to reach
the flat cutting line. With
this way of shaping the
hair, those shorter hairs
blend in very well.

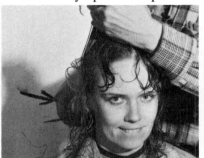
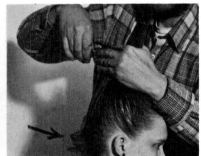

● When you gave the equal-length cut, you were cautioned about trying
to get too much hair into your HGH grasp. The length and amount of
hair being combed up around the sides and back on this haircut is such
that you can't be concerned about this "overloading" problem—the
unevenness that results from this is smoothed off later.

● The haircuttee's head gets moved around.
You always have to move the haircuttee's
head around during any haircut to achieve
easy comb-handling and maximum vision.
This haircut requires more than the usual
head-bending cooperation as you comb up
the hair around the sides and back.

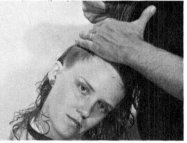

● On the equal-length cut, you combed the sides and back hair down
before beginning a pathway up through the hair. On this cut, the more
the hair can stay combed up after a comb up and cut, the easier it is.

4. The Sequence of Pathways Around the Head

This is the way you'll
work around the head.
One long comb up and
cut takes care of each
path.

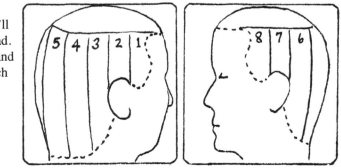

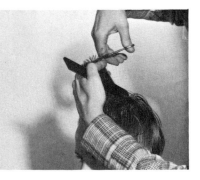

Pathway 1 The first comb up and cut off is done to the same front right-side pathway you used on the equal-length haircut's right section.

After you have made this first cut, the rest of the pathways you comb up and cut will have an extra guide-hair aid to rely on. In addition to combing the hair up so that you include some cut hair from the top section, you also **overlap** the comb up so you include 1/2 inch or more of the pathway that has just been combed up and cut.

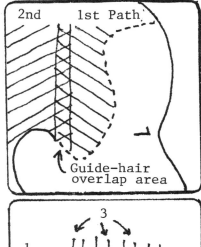

As you see, on the second pathway's comb up and cut, the extra guide-hair comes from where your second path overlaps the first path. You will be able to employ this extra help on the second path, and on all the rest of the pathways around the head.

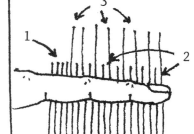

When you carefully comb up the hair on the second pathway, the hair between your holding fingers will include (1) guide-hair from the overlap area, (2) guide-hair from the already-cut top section, (3) hairs to be cut.

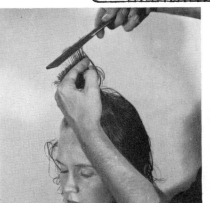
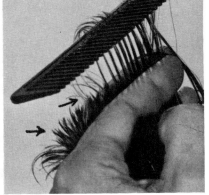

This photo and the blow-up clearly show the double guide-hair. The arrows point to the guide-hair from the side's first pathway and the guide-hair from the top section.

The reason for overlapping the paths is that it insures **all** the hair long enough to reach to the top is cut—you can't miss a hair.

* * *

Cross a porcupine with a gorilla and whatever it is will sure get a seat on a bus.

George Carlin

<u>Pathways 2 – 8</u> The first pathway's comb up and cut was shown on the previous page. Here we continue the trip around the head.

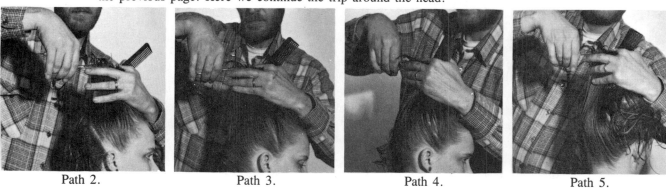

Path 2.   Path 3.   Path 4.   Path 5.

Step over to the haircuttee's right and finish your cuts.

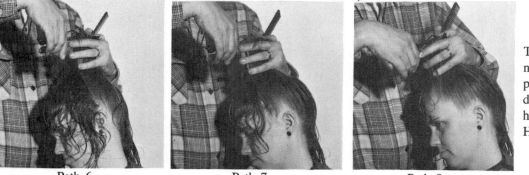

Path 6.   Path 7.   Path 8.

The exact number of paths will depend on head and HGH size.

Now go back to path 1, and do your second-time-through cutting by repeating all of the cuts around the head. Cut off only the stragglers.

D. Smoothing Off

When you are finished with the top and sides/back parts of the bulk-removal, you'll find a little unevenness where these two parts of your cutting meet.

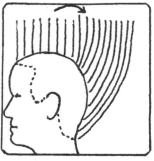
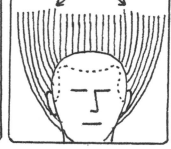

To deal with this unevenness, you go through the same pathways 4 and 5 used on the equal-length haircut's top section. Here the comb is handled in a different way than was used on the equal-length cut: once the comb is positioned flat to the scalp (teeth scraping the scalp), you lift the comb in a **pivoting** manner like this on pathway 4.

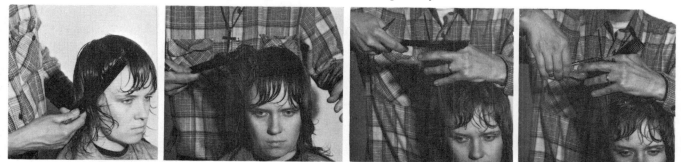

Do this cutting with the haircuttee on a high chair.

Use the comb-away method as you comb up for the cuts in pathway 5. Keep in mind your flat cutting line and place the top of your holding fingers just below it.

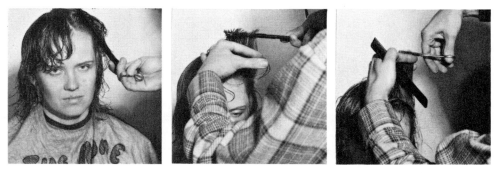

This smooth off cutting has a more familiar double guide-hair aid to use. The hair to be cut appears like this:

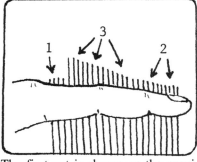

1. At the "V" of the fingers you'll have the already-cut, top section hair to use as a guide.
2. Out at the finger tips are the hair ends from the sides that you'll use as a second guide.
3. The hair between the two guides will be cut off.

The first cut is shown on the previous page. The rest of pathway 4 goes like this:

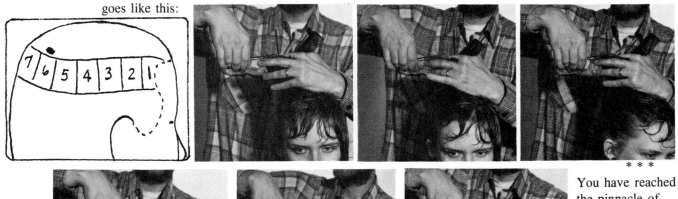

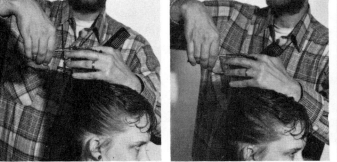

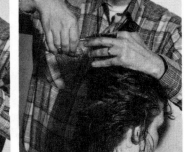

* * *

You have reached the pinnacle of success as soon as you become uninterested in money, compliments, or publicity.
Dr.O.A. Battista

Finish pathway 5 using the comb-away (the first cut is shown above).

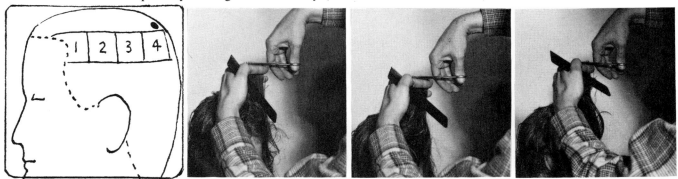

9.5 EDGE-CUTTING

The edge-cutting for the long, layered cut differs significantly from
the way it was done on the equal-length cut.

A. Methods You'll Use

While the equal-length and short, full cuts need a variety of
edge cutting techniques to trim those perimeter hairs evenly, with the
long, layered cut you can use just the pull-and-cut method. (Force of
habit usually has me using the modified-bulk-removal technique on the
bangs and temple region hair, but it's not necessary.)

B. Shape of the Cutting Line

When you did the edging on the equal-length cut, the hair was combed
straight out from the hairline and cut so the edgeline was, by and
large, equal distance from the hairline. With our long cut you also
comb the hair fairly straight out and away from the hairline to make
the cuts, but because of the increasing length of the hair, you cut
the edgeline so it **conforms** to this increasing length of the hair
around the sides.

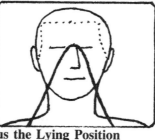

To get this cutting to go
along with the bulk-cutting,
you must do the edging
around the face in the
shape of a Christmas tree.

This tree shape is
achieved, snip-by-snip,
while the top and side
hair is combed forward
and held toward the
lower part of the face.

C. The Cutting Position Versus the Lying Position

Back in chapter 6, I explained how the final lying position for the
edge hair would shrink up, and be shorter than the hair is while being
cut. This rule of haircutting is even more noticeable when you do the
edging on the long, layered cut, especially if the hair has a Type 2
grain or if it's wavy or curly. Straighter types of hair with a Type 1
hairgrain are not affected by this shrinking edgeline as much; but, to
be on the safe side, you should make your edge cuts at least 2 inches
longer than the lying position you want for the edge hair. Curlier
hair or hair with a Type 2 grain needs as much as 4 inches of extra
length. You can always cut off more later, but once it is gone, . . .

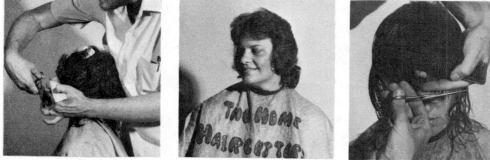

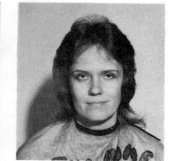

Cutting versus lying position.   Cutting versus lying position.

You'll find the difference between the position of the cutting line
and the final lying position is especially noticeable on the hair that
frames the face—that hair normally lies toward the back of the head,
but the cutting is done with the hair pulled forward.

D. How It's Done

Cutting the long, layered cut's edgeline just requires an awareness of the Christmas tree shape you strive for. You cut with this shape in mind while the hair is pulled forward in the general direction of the lower half of the center of the face.

1. **Sequence of Cuts**. The preliminary or final edging for the long, layered cut always starts at the top of the tree and proceeds down the person's right side to the longest hair at the back of the head. Then back to the tree-top and down and around the left side.

Remember, when you do the bulk-cutting for this haircut (as with the other two kinds of cuts), you already have the edge hairs cut and in the basic shape you want—when doing the final edging you only cut off a **little** unevenness. This sequence of cuts allows you to comb a little of the already-cut edgeline hair into your HGH grasp on each cut you make after the first one. Be sure to use that guide-hair.

Starting at the top of the tree, you stand at a 12 – 1 o'clock position for the pull-and-cut, or a 3 – 4 o'clock spot for the modified-bulk-removal. Assuming your top center path was cut to the recommended 3 inch length and your haircuttee has an average hairline in front, the hair at the tree-top will lie at the bridge of the nose. Comb the hair to be cut from the crown region to the edges where your HGH waits to grasp the hair—use this lengthy combing for each cut.

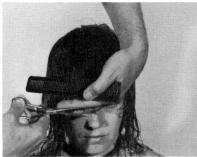 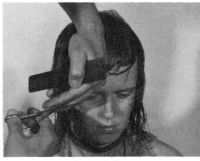 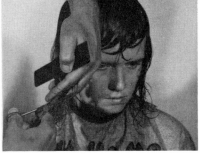

Cut 1.   Cut 2.   Cut 3.

After you cut the upper part of the tree on the haircuttee's right side, use the pull-and-cut on the rest of the cuts you make on the trip to the middle of the back hair. The following photos show the cutting done above the holding fingers: remember to do your cutting the preferred, safer way with the cuts made on the **inside** of the fingers.

For these cuts you want to have a straight-on line of vision. The haircuttee sits on a high chair or both you and the haircuttee stand.

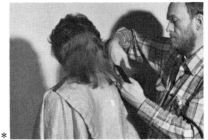

* * *

Love for one's country which is not part of one's love for humanity is not love, but idolatrous worship.   Erich Fromm
A foul mouth is the voice of a polluted soul.   Anonymous
Racism is a social disease.   Message on a button
Sexism is a social disease.   Message on a button
Porn is the theory, rape is the practice.   Message on a button
No doubt Jack the Ripper excused himself on the grounds that it was human nature.   A. A. Milne
Never in this world can hatred be stilled by hatred; it will be stilled only by non-hatred—this is the law eternal.   Buddha
It is possible to live in peace.   Mohandas Gandhi

You cut your way to the back.

Return to the front and the top of the tree.

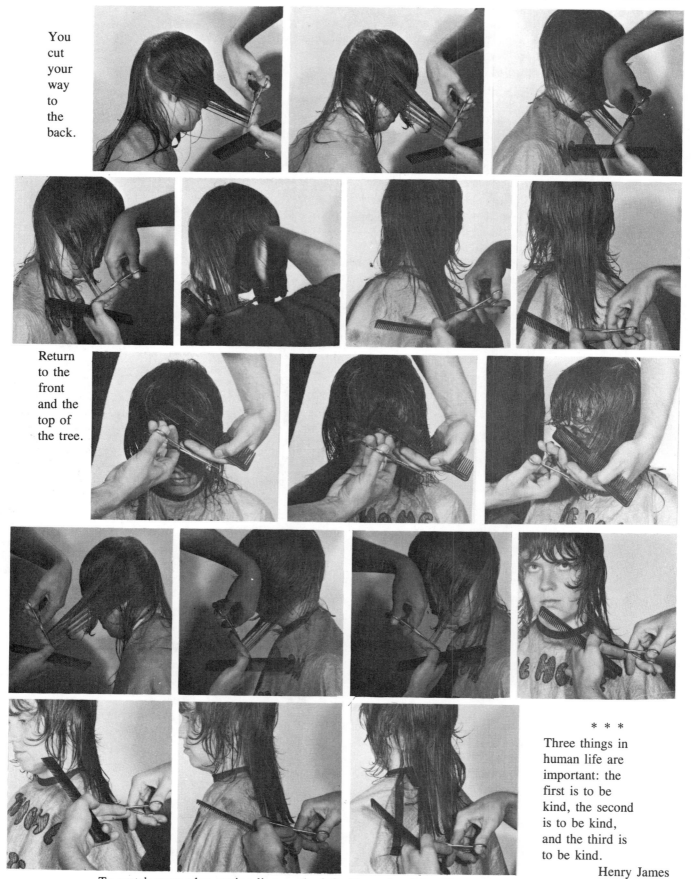

* * *

Three things in human life are important: the first is to be kind, the second is to be kind, and the third is to be kind.

Henry James

To match your edge-cutting line on the left side to the right side,

you must do the following:
- Remember, cut off a minimum of hair and use that guide-hair.
- Keep a mental picture of where your HGH was positioned on the right side in relation to the features of the face (nose, mouth, chin, neck) and duplicate those positions on the left.
- If one side is a little shorter than the other when the hair is in its normal lying state, trim the longer side to match the shorter.

2. **Side Part**. Flat shaping and Christmas tree edging works well if the hair has a center or somewhat off-center part. If the hairgrain dictates a side part, the umbrella version of a long, layered cut or the combination cut (see sections 6-B and C in this chapter) are well-suited, but they are the shortest of the long cuts—maybe too short for your haircuttee. If you give the flat shaped version to hair with a side part, the Christmas tree edging is done as previously shown, then make some modifications:
- Find the natural part and comb the top toward its preferred lying side.

- Trim that portion of the bangs closest to the part so those hairs are as short as the top of the tree hairs.

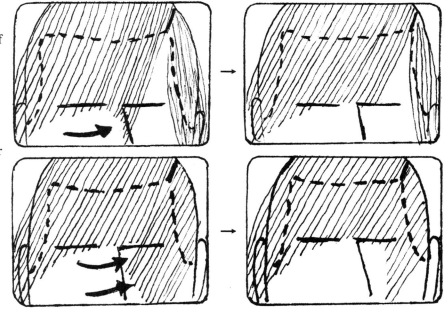

- Then trim the upper temple region hairs a little so they blend with the shorter bangs hair. Trimming the first few inches of the upper side hair will remove the unevenness.

9.6 MODIFYING THE LONG, LAYERED CUT

These ways to modify a long, layered cut are arranged from the easiest to the more difficult. While the first option can be used with your initial haircuts, I don't recommend the others until you're comfortable with the haircut shown in the cut-by-cut photos.

A. A Shorter Overall Length

The length you leave the hair on the top pathways determines the overall length of a long, layered haircut. This is due to the way the sides and back are pulled up and cut while using the top hair as a guide for how much is cut off. A shorter cutting on top leaves all the hair shorter; a longer cutting on top leaves all the hair longer.

A shorter cutting on top doesn't require any changes from how you did the bulk-removal for the longer cut shown earlier. A flat cutting is still the goal, the only difference is a shorter length-producing position for your holding-guide-hand (HGH) while cutting the top. This shorter cutting may allow you to rest the bottom of your HGH on the scalp while cutting the top section's second and third paths, and as you pull up the sides and back hair for cutting.

Because of the shorter length, your edge-cutting line is altered to some extent. The Christman tree edge-line needs to be higher on the forehead, and wider at the top.

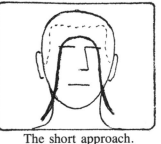
The short approach.

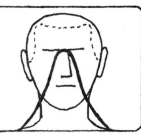
A longer cutting.

This shorter cutting is well-suited to fine hair, or the wavier, curly, and kinky types of hair. The finer or curlier the hair, the shorter it can be cut: you can go as short as 1 inch on the first path, but 1 1/2 – 2 inches usually works best. (If the hair is cut extra short and you want to leave the bangs longer, refer back to pages 117 and 118 for the how-to.) Keep in mind: straight, coarse-textured hair may not lie well if cut shorter than 3 inches.

B. Umbrella Shape

This way to shape hair, when combined with a shorter cutting on top, produces the shortest version of the long, layered cut.

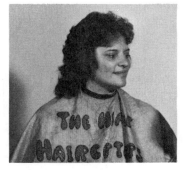

* * *

You may speak of love, tenderness, and passion, but for real ecstasy discover that you haven't lost your keys after all.
Anonymous

If you lend a friend money and you never see him again, it's worth it.
Anonymous

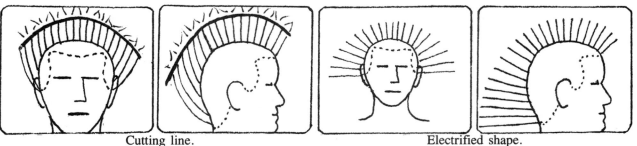
Cutting line.   Electrified shape.

1. Bulk-Removal

This haircut's top 3 paths are done the same way as the equal-length cut's first 3 paths: the holding fingers conform to the head's shape. With every head somewhat rounded on top, when you begin with an equal-length cutting on the top 3 pathways, you create a rounded cutting line. The cutting line on the sides and back is a fairly straight line that slopes downward—it's a continuation of the cutting line established on the top 3 pathways. Because of this, the shape of the top of the head does affect the overall cutting line.

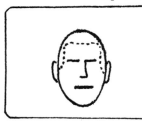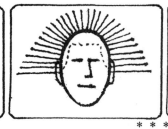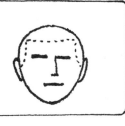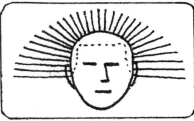

* * *

If life hands you a lemon—make lemonade!   Anonymous
There is nothing like sealing a letter to inspire a fresh thought.
Anonymous

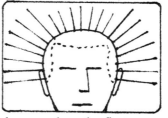

Part 1 Cut the top three paths with the holding fingers conforming to the shape of the head. After you have finished these paths, the electrified shape would show unevenness. The next part removes this unevenness and shapes the rest of the hair.

Part 2 Follow the same pathways and long comb up used on the first long cut's sides and back hair. Due to the equal-length cutting on the top three paths, you'll be able to rest the bottom of your HGH on the scalp, instead of holding it out in space.

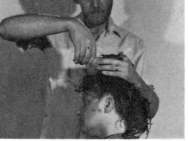

Now the bottom of the HGH can rest on the head.

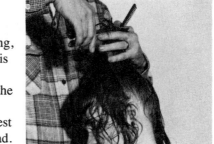

With flat line shaping, the HGH is floating, and only the wrist or forearm rest on the head.

Part 3 Use the same "pivoting" comb manipulation and the same pathways you used for the smooth off cuts on the flat shaping. After you cut pathways 4 and 5, additional pathways 6 and 7 (just below and parallel to 4 and 5) may also be necessary. This cutting has your holding fingers sloped downward instead of being held straight out as they were for the flat cut. Rest your HGH or wrist on the top side of the head.

With this cutting, like the smooth off cuts on the flat shaping, you remove only a little unevenness that results from the part 1 and part 2 cutting.

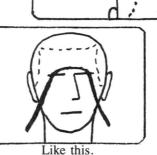

2. Edging

The edging shape for this cut reflects the shorter bulk-removal on the sides of the top section. Here your Christmas tree gets fatter.

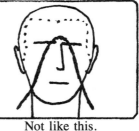

Like this.   Not like this.

This version of the long cut works well with any hair, but it's extra well-suited to curlier hair, and fine hair with a Type 2 hairgrain.

C. Combination Cut

This long haircut's bulk-removal is a mixture of an equal-length cut and a long, layered cut; if you choose an edging treatment to the hair around the ears like that shown in the example, your combination cut borrows something from all three basic haircuts. This way to shape the hair has the extra easy-care features of the shorter equal-length haircut, and some of the longer appearance of the long, layered cut.

* * *

Work is love made visible.   Anonymous
Generous people are rarely mentally ill.   Dr. Karl Menninger

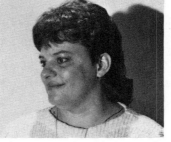
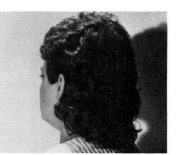

The combination cut is similar to the equal-length cut that has the back hair shaped longer. But there are some new "twists" to this cutting, and the overall appearance is considerably longer:

1. Bulk-Removal

The bulk-cutting consists of two main parts and a third smooth off cutting.

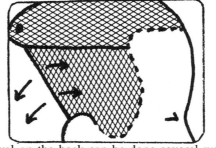

Part 1 First give an equal-length cutting (2 – 3 inches) to the top section, and to this portion of the side section:

For the side cutting, you need to part the hair from the rear upper ear to the crown region.

Part 2 The bulk-removal on the back can be done several ways—the longer cutting approaches are extra adaptable to straighter hair, the shorter approaches work on any type of hair, but especially curlier hair. These options are arranged from longest to shortest:

● Pathway by pathway, pull up and cut off the back section hair as you did for the flat shaping of the long, layered cut.

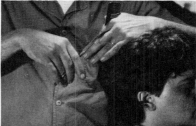

● Make a path around the upper 2 – 3 inches of the back so it has a gradually increasing length—the same way it's done for the umbrella version. Then pull up the back hair (pathway by pathway) to the bottom of this path and cut off the excess back length.

● Repeat the second option, but make one more path just below and parallel to the path around the upper back. Pull up the lower back hair and cut it while using the bottom of this second path as a guide for how much is cut off.

Part 3 The area where you go from an equal-length cutting on the sides to the increasing length around the upper back needs more than the usual smoothing off cuts to make it blend together. This area needs the holding fingers positioned so they go along with the increased length on the back hair, while you also have some of the shorter side hair in your grasp.

This cutting can be done with a horizontal HGH positioning while standing at the opposite side of the head. However, it may be easier to employ the cutting technique used for approximate bulk-cutting (see page 68). This method has you stand on the same side you're working on. One path should do it, but two might be needed if the back hair was given one of the longer length-producing options.

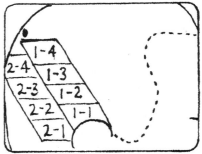

2. Edging

Cut the bangs and temple area as you did for the equal-length cut. The edging on the hair around the ears can be done so some part of the ear

is left covered, or it can be cut so all of the ear shows (most prefer
this second option). Whichever option you choose, don't cut any of the
longer hair at the upper, back part of the ear. To explain how you go
about it, both types of hairgrain have to be looked at.

● **Type 2 hairgrain.** Assume the bulk-cutting left the side hair
2 1/2 inches.

If you want to
leave some of the
ear covered, you
can give it a
straight-across
edging line as
used on the
equal-length cut.

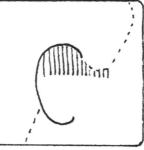

Or the edging
line can follow
the hairline
above, and in
front of the
ear.

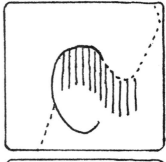

If all the ear is
to be exposed, comb
the side hair down,
over the ear and
cut off 1 – 1 1/2
inches of length so
the edgeline
conforms to hair-
line above and in
front of the ear.

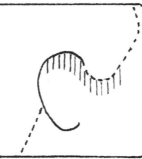

Comb side hair
back—it rises
up and sits on
top of the ear.
The hair at the
dip (in front
of ear) can be
cut as shown
here, or it can
be left as is.

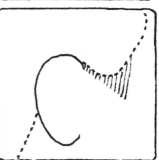

● **Type 1 hairgrain.** With the hair growing straight down, you need
to leave the hair longer to have it bend toward the back (the way most
people like to wear this haircut). Again, we'll assume 2 1/2 inches of
length from the bulk-cutting (3 inches maybe needed on coarser hair).
If the side hair is to lie toward the back, give the edge hairs a
minimum cutting with the edgeline conforming to the hairline, from the
dip to the top back of the ear. If the side hair is to lie downward,
the edgeline can be cut as short as you want—most prefer the
straight-across cutting line.

With either hairgrain type, if you cut off 1 – 2 inches of the
bottom side hair, you will need to taper that bottom hair a little.
(See the 2-step tapering method in the previous chapter.)

The edging that starts at the top, back of the ear and goes down
the side of the neck is done much the same as you did it for an
equal-length haircut with longer neck hair—the extra length of the
back hair means your edging line is more toward the face. You want
this edging to be a minimum cut-off that reflects the increasing
length of the back hair. Don't attempt to blend the shorter hair from
above the ear with the longer hair from the back—just pull that
longer back hair forward and ignore the shorter hair. Do the edging on
the back, bottom hair using the pull-and-cut. Most prefer this hair to
be quite long, but it can be cut shorter than the minimum cut-off used
on the side of the neck. After you've cut across the bottom, round off
the corners where the bottom meets the sides of the neck.

The combination cut is adaptable to any hair, but it's extra good
for wavy or curly types of hair, or finer-textured straight hair with
a Type 2 grain—the kind that flips forward in the lower temple area
if left too long (page 173 has more on this condition).

D. An Extra Long Version

As explained earlier, the overall length of a long, layered cut depends on the length of the top hair. This longest of the long haircuts is saved for last because the extra length on top means your HGH won't have anything to rest on during the bulk-removal—your hands float in space and your arms get extra tired.

The bulk-removal for this version is cut the same as for the basic long, layered haircut. The edge cutting-line is altered to conform to the longer bulk-cutting.

The Christmas tree's top is lower and the overall shape is skinnier than the shorter versions.

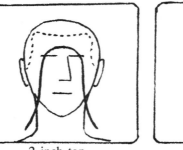
2 inch top.

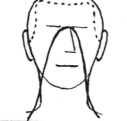
3 inch top.

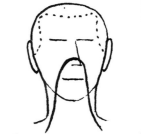
5 inch top.

The first of the three pathways on top can be left as long as 6 – 7 inches, but as this photo shows, 5 inches on the beginning path leaves plenty of extra length.

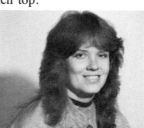

This longer cutting can be used with any hair; however, wavy hair or coarse, straight hair works best.

While this is the most challenging of the long haircuts, when you're comfortable with the earlier versions, you should be in good shape to handle it.

9.7 CHECK FOR LENGTH EVENNESS

You easily checked the equal-length cut for consistent length by randomly pulling the hair straight out from the head in 10 – 12 places and measuring that hair with a ruler. With the increasing lengths of long, layered cuts, you have to be exacting in where you do your checking. The parts of the head to be checked include the following:
● Sides. If you pick a checkpoint, say 2 inches above the ear, be sure to check the exact same spot on the other side.
● Top left checking requires a corresponding spot on the top right.
● Back section—left side versus the right side. Measure at points that are the same distance up from the hairline at both checkpoints.

With this kind of haircut the tendency is to gradually leave the hair too long during the bulk-removal. For example, the first side (right) of the haircuttee's head is cut to the correct length, but by the time you get around to the left side, your holding-guide-hand (HGH) has left the hair longer and longer.

If you find an area longer than its counterpart on the other side of the head or section, go to the area that is shorter and check your HGH position when the hair is held in the cutting position: back to the longer area to recut with the correct HGH position duplicated there.

When you have these ways of shaping hair in your bag of skills, you are ready for the last, most challenging of the three basic haircuts.

* * *

A job is the self-portrait of the person that did it.   Anonymous

10.1 INTRODUCTION

To round-off your skills development, you need to know about short haircutting. The cut-by-cut part of the chapter teaches a short, full haircut and the new ways to manipulate your hands. This somewhat longer (more full) version of a short haircut was chosen because it can be cut with just scissors and comb (no clippers needed), and because of its popularity. The later pages show some variations of our main short haircut.

    As these before-and-after photos show, the final appearance of short, full cuts differs about as much as the different hair qualities each of these folks have.

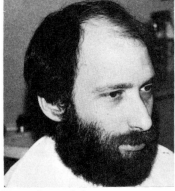

Type 1, straight, medium texture. Thinning top needs shorter length.

Top is cut to 1 3/4 inches; 3/4 inch around bottoms.

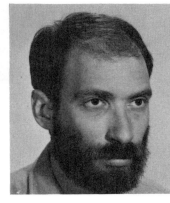

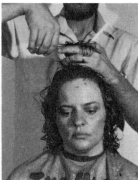

Type 2, extra wavy, medium texture.

3 inch length on top; 1 inch around bottoms— shorter in front of ears. Bangs cut shorter than minimum cutting.

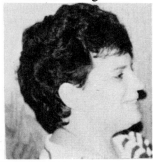

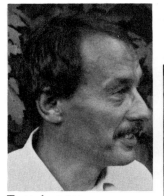

Type 1, extra fine, straight hair.

Top is cut to 1 1/2 inches; 3/4 inch around the bottoms

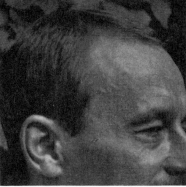

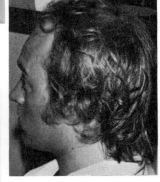

Type 1 (lower temple grows toward back), fine, slightly wavy. Short growing hair around bottoms.

Cut to 1 3/4 inches on top; a little less than 3/4 inch around bottoms.

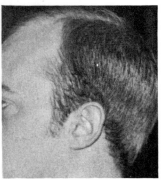

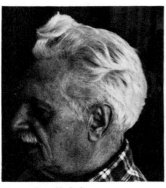

Type 2, slightly
wavy, medium
texture.

Top is cut to
1 3/4 inches;
3/4 inch around
bottoms.

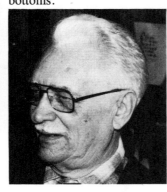

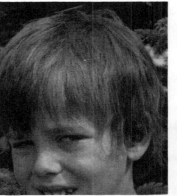

Type 1, straight,
medium texture.
Cowlick on front
hairline needs
extra top length.

Top is 2 1/2
inches with
bangs trimmed
shorter than
minimum cutting;
3/4 inch around
bottoms.

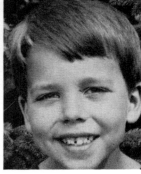

This shortest way to shape hair is taught last because it is the most
difficult of the three haircuts. There are two main reasons why this
is such a challenging haircut:

● Because of the shortness of this cut, your cutting has to be extra
precise. With a 2 – 3 inch equal-length cut, you can leave the hair
with unevenness (as much as a 1/4 inch, even as much as 1/2 inch on
curlier hair) and it won't show—you still have a well done haircut.
The long, layered cut gives you even more room for error. With the
short, full haircut, **any** unevenness sticks out like a sore thumb.
A cooperative haircuttee who can hold their head still, and a very
precise use of the HGH is needed for success on this haircut.

● You will be tapering in a decreasing length to
the hair around the sides and back. This tapering
would be simple if a head of hair had the growing
surface shown here. However, a typical head of
hair has about 2 1/2 – 3 inches of growing surface
on the sides and about 5 – 6 inches on the back.

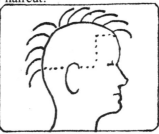

Because of the equal-length cutting on the top section, you begin your
tapering with the same length (for example, 2 inches) all around the
upper sides and back, and you gradually taper the length on the sides
and back until the bottom hair, all around the head, is cut to a
length of 3/4 inch or a little less. The difficulty arises because the
back section has twice as much distance to achieve this tapering, as
do the sides: you must **blend** together the tapering on the 3 inch-
long side sections and the 6 inch-long back section so that it's all
smoothly cut, uniformly graduated. Difficult? Yes! Take longer to do?
For sure. But with the experience you have from the first two cuts and
the how-to directions here, you can expect to produce the type of
excellent short cuts given by better professionals.

10.2 BULK-REMOVAL

A. Top Section

Short haircuts generally need the top hair cut on the shorter side
(2 1/2 inches or less) to have the whole head of hair fit together—so
the top is in balance with the shortness around the lower portions of

the hair. The top five pathways are cut as if you were giving an
equal-length haircut. (Page 161 shows how to do it if the top hair is
left longer than 2 1/2 inches.)

B. **Sides and Back**

There are a number of ways to do the tapered cutting needed for this
part of the haircut—the photos show my preferred method (see page 160
for other ways).

    This haircut, more than the first two, needs you to clearly
visualize the cutting line and shape you want because your holding-
guide-hand (HGH) gets into a variety of positions that produce a
gradually decreasing length. Your HGH conforms to the shape of this
cutting line as the hair is held **straight** out from the head. (See
chapter 3, page 46 to review the cutting line for this haircut.)

Pathway 1 This path is just below and parallel to pathway 4 on the
top section. The first few cuts in this right side pathway are
slightly tapered.

For example, the top is cut to a 2 inch
length. Position your HGH so that you
leave the hair 2 inches long at the "V"
of the holding fingers, and a bit more
than 1 1/2 inches at the finger tips.
Use the 2 inch long hair from the
already-cut top section as guide-hair:
it appears at the "V".

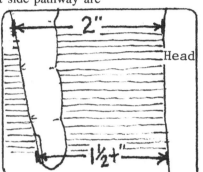

Here is the way it goes:

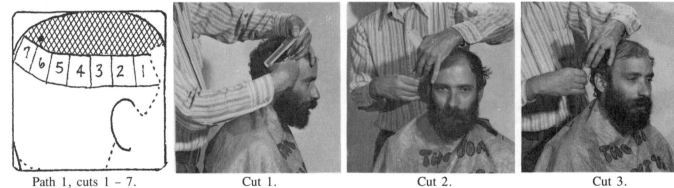

Path 1, cuts 1 – 7.   Cut 1.   Cut 2.   Cut 3.

To accomodate the back section and its 6 inch-long growing surface,
use an equal-length HGH positioning as you do the rest of the path
around the back of the head.

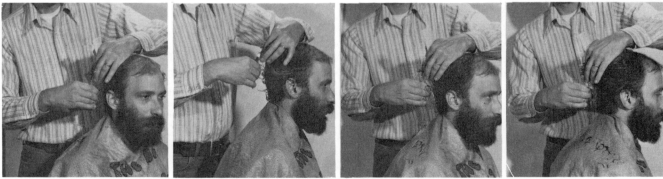

Cut 4.   Cut 5.   Cut 6.   Cut 7.

With a Type 1 hairgrain, the sequence of cuts shown above works well.
If you have a Type 2 grain to work with, you may have to reverse the

sequence of cuts: start at the back of the head and proceed to the front right side while using the comb-away method.

Remember, before you begin cutting, comb the hair in the opposite direction from your travel through the path. Here the hair was combed toward the front before this pathway cutting began.

Pathway 2 Again, the first three cuts are slightly tapered; then you resume an equal-length cutting for the rest of the path. Use the comb-away method. Type 2 hairgrain may need the basic manipulation starting at the back and working your way to the front. The guide-hair from the top section is at the "V" of the holding fingers.

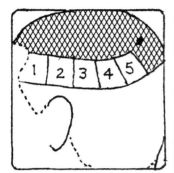

Path 2, cuts 1 – 5.

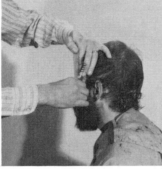

Cut 1.

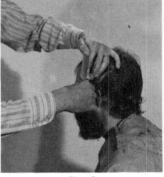

Cut 2.

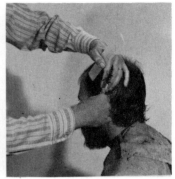

Cut 3.

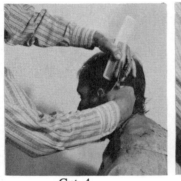

Cut 4.

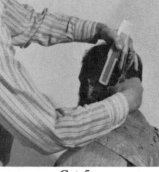

Cut 5.

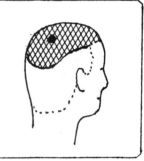

At this point you have tapered the upper sides a little, and the checkered portion has an equal-length cutting.

Now, back to the right side for some "heavy duty" tapering. . . .

Pathway 3 To do this cutting you manipulate the HGH as you did for 2-step tapering of neck hair (shown on page 115). Use the diagonal HGH positioning, but now the holding finger tips **touch** the skin—this cutting is done to the hair beginning at the hairline and above, whereas the tapering you did on the neck hair was concerned with longer hairs 1 – 2 inches above the neck's edgeline. Your finger tips can't touch the skin on the first cut because of the sideburn, but it can for the rest of the cuts. Your holding fingers curve away from the scalp, up to and including the cut hair from the first pathway on the right side—use that guide-hair found at the "V".

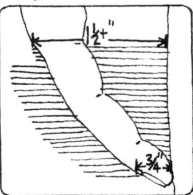

Start at a 4 – 5 o'clock position and move to 9 – 10 o'clock as you work around the head. The pathway illustration had to be "distorted" a little to show all the cuts you make in this trip around the bottom.

* * *

My belief is that to have no wants is divine.   Socrates

Idealists . . . foolish enough to throw caution to the winds . . . have advanced mankind and have enriched the world.   Emma Goldberg

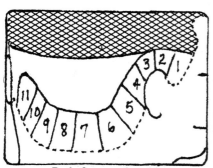

Path 3, cuts 1 – 11.

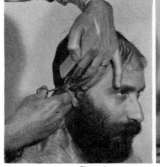

Cut 1.

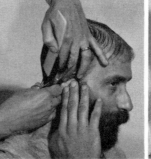

Cut 2.

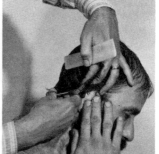

Cut 3.

At about this point, you get away from the neighboring pathway
approach as you continue down the neck and around the bottom of the
back. You won't have any guide-hair to use, so be careful to keep the
exact same out-and-away (curved) HGH position for the remaining
cuts, as those used on the first three cuts.

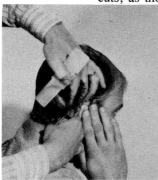

Cut 4.

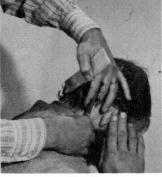

Cut 5.

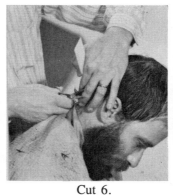

Cut 6.

Cut 7.

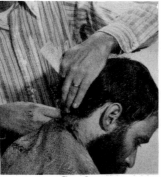

Cut 8.

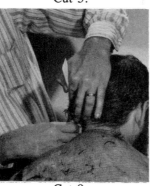

Cut 9.

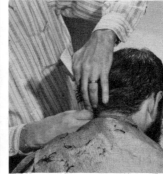

Cut 10.

Cut 11.

If the hair has a ducktail neckline and a strong Type 2 hairgrain, you
may need to start this path at the tail and travel around the bottom
to the front right side, while using the comb-away method. Then return
to the ducktail and do cuts 8 – 11 shown above.

Pathway 4 Cutting this path between the two already-cut paths
around the back is the best way to get the long, **gradual** tapering
that is needed for the back of the head.

You don't
want this
to happen.

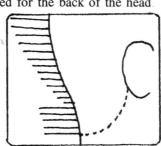

You want this—it's
much easier to
achieve when done
as shown.

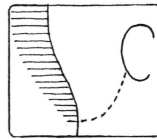

As the photos below show, this path between the two cut paths has double guide-hair to use (at the "V" and finger tips). Keep your holding fingers fairly straight, and cut all the hair between the two guides.

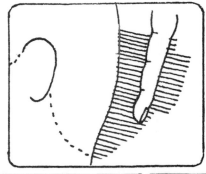

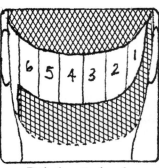

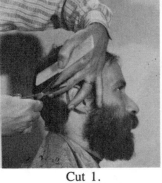

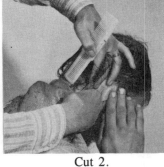

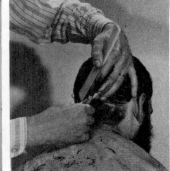

Path 4, cuts 1 – 6.   Cut 1.   Cut 2.   Cut 3.

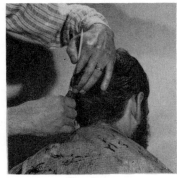

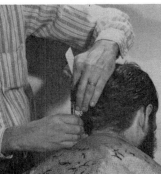

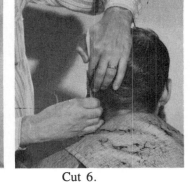

Depending on head and HGH size, you may have to make an additional path above this one.

Cut 4.   Cut 5.   Cut 6.

Pathway 5 This last path has you return to the same "heavy" tapering that was done to the right side and back. You have guide-hair at the "V" again. The finger tips rest on the skin, right at the hairline.

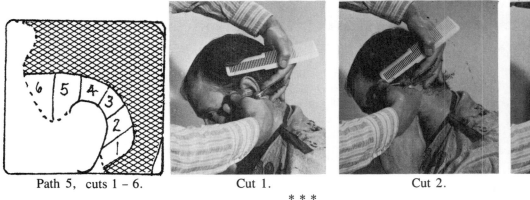

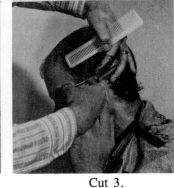

Path 5, cuts 1 – 6.   Cut 1.   Cut 2.   Cut 3.

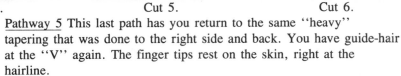

* * *

Since the beginning of time each generation has fought nature. Now in the span of a single generation, we must turn and become the protector of nature.   Jacques Cousteau

Those who speak most of progress measure it by quantity and not by quality.   George Santayana

Economic growth is not only unnecessary, but ruinous.   A. Solzhenitsyn

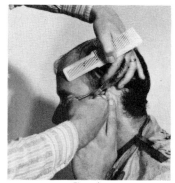
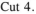

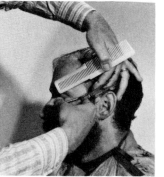

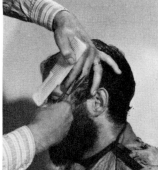

Cut 4.   Cut 5.   Cut 6.

In cutting this path, it doesn't matter if the hair has Type 1 or 2 grain—this sequence of cuts works well with either.

10.3 SMOOTHING OFF

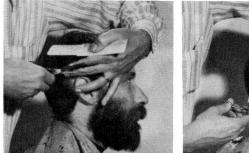

For this second-time-through cutting, you go through the hair with the HGH held in an opposite position from what was used during the first-time-through. Here you position the holding fingers horizontally, instead of vertically or diagonally.

Before we start cutting, you should be aware of the following:

● The first-time-through bulk-removal usually leaves a little more unevenness than what you are used to, especially in this area on each side of the head:

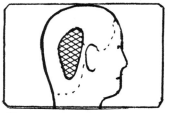

This unevenness is a result of going from the three-inch long sides to the six-inch long back section hair. This second-time-through cutting gets these areas smoothly-cut.

● For the second cutting, you start at the bottom of the sides and back, and move up through pathways from there. Because most of your tapering occurred on the bottom 2 – 3 inches around the head, each pathway up the head needs the stepping-out method (see pages 116 and 117) for the first several manipulations you make up the path.

● How far away from the scalp you position your holding fingers for each manipulation was determined solely by the cutting done on the first-time-through bulk-removal. For example, the first cut in any pathway is always at the hairline: here your holding fingers touch the skin. They are in the shortest possible cutting position because your finger tips touched the skin when you did the first-time-through on the bottom path.

The hair between the holding fingers will look something like this:

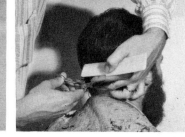

Cut off only the longer hair— the shorter hair is your guide-hair.

* * *

I am never bored anywhere: being bored is an insult to oneself.   Renard

Because of the increasing length the higher into the
pathway you go, when you repeat the next manipulation
one inch up from the first one, you'll have longer
hair protruding from the holding fingers. To smooth
off these hairs, slide your HGH out on the hairshafts
so you have the same amount of guide-hair sticking
out (1/8 – 1/4 inch) from the holding fingers as is
shown at the bottom of the previous page.

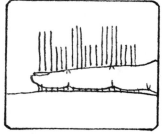

Cut off those longer hairs and your smooth it off goal is realized.
When the stepping-out cuts are done this way, the cuts always conform
to and blend with the tapering you achieved on the bulk-removal.

A. Sequence of Paths

1. **Right side**. Your first pathway starts at the bottom of the
front right side, near the sideburn, and proceeds up to the top-front-
center of the hairline.

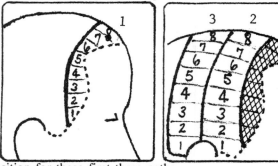

Some manipulations will have
you hold and cut small amounts
of hair. That's fine—you want
to establish a straight path
for the next pathways to
follow. Paths 2 and 3 are
alongside the first path.

Stand at the 8 – 10:00 o'clock position for these first three paths.
Seat your haircuttee on a low chair, and you'll need more than the
usual amount of head-bending cooperation.

Your next 2 pathways are on
the side of the neck. These
short paths are straight-away
from the hairline. Stand at
6 – 7 o'clock and expect to
need some ear folding help.

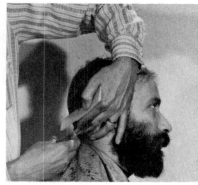

After you have finished the
the short paths, make two
paths up to the rear part of
the top of the head—they
begin where the two short
paths left off.

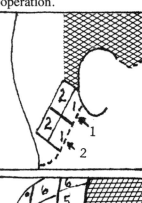

* * *

Men once subscribed to
the theory of male
superiority, but women
have cancelled the
subscription.   Anon.
Feminists just want
the human race to be a
tie.   Anonymous

2. **Back section**. For the back of the head, follow the same
pathways and sequence of cuts used during the bulk-removal on the
equal-length cut (see chapter 8, section 4-C). The first pathway on
this back section has you go back over part of the area you worked on
during the side of the neck cutting. Good! This area is where you find
most of the unevenness in a short, full cut—it can stand an extra
going over.

3. **Left side**. The first 2 paths are the same as the paths on the
right side, except that here you reverse the sequence of short paths,
and your holding fingers point in an upward direction instead of
downwards. Keep standing at 4 – 5 o'clock for the 2 longer paths that
go up to the top. (Again, you are going over the last path from the
back section—this area needs it.) Finish your smooth off efforts with
the 3 front side paths, beginning where your last cutting left off.

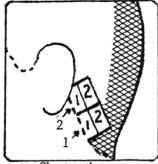
Short paths.

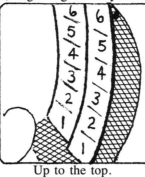
Up to the top.

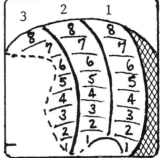
The last paths.

* * *
A banker is a
fellow who
hands you an
umbrella when
the sun is
shining and
wants it back
the minute it
begins to rain.
Mark Twain

At this point, your precision-cut short, full haircut is almost
completed. Before you do the edging, dry the hair and inspect it for
heavy spots or cutting lines. Once more, go through the trouble spots
behind and above the ears—trim as needed for maximum smoothness.

10.4 EDGING

After you do the bulk-cutting for short haircuts (like the other two
you've learned), the edgeline is close to the way you want it. Just
cutting a few stragglers is all that should be needed.

A. Sequence to Follow
1. **Bangs**. Because the top hair was cut to the same length, use
the same methods here as used for the equal-length cut.
2. **Upper right temple region**. The questions of whether to trim and
what methods to use are the same for this cut as for the equal-length
cut (see pages 122 and 123).
3. **Lower temple**. Because of the tapered cutting around the lower
sides, your edging also has a decreasing length. Before you cut, comb
the hair back to see the shape of the hairline. Then comb the hair
toward the front and use the finger-bracing or the scissors-and-comb
method (or both).
Give the lower temple
region this kind of
decreasing length on
the edgeline. This
has the edge cuts
conforming to the
bulk-removal tapering.

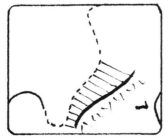

* * *
Remember, it's only from the
valley that the mountain
seems so high.   Anonymous
A journey of a thousand miles
begins with just one step.
Anonymous

4. **Right sideburn**. Use the same methods here as you used when
sideburn cutting on the equal-length cut.
5. **Right side**. With the short cut you are limited in the edging
methods that can be used because of the length of the hair. Comb the
hair straight away from the hairline and use the finger-bracing
method. If you are working on Type 2 hairgrain, you may have to use
the scissors-and-comb method to get the hair straight out from the
hairline—particularily above and behind the ear.

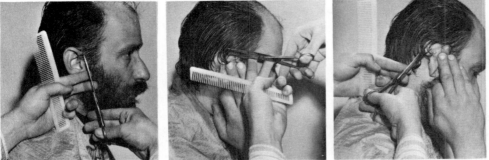

Any part of this edging may require you to reverse the direction the scissors takes. Do whatever is easiest and most effective.

On a Type 2 grain, the cutting path should begin at the bottom of the neck and go upward over the ear (pages 80 and 81 explained why).

6. **Neckline**. Use the finger-bracing method to cut a straight line across the back. Be sure the line is at or below the hairline.

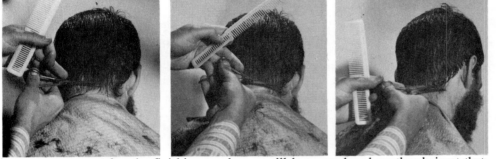

After you round off the corner where the right side of the neck and the bottom neckline meet, go to the left temple and work your way to the back on the "port" side.

After the finishing touches, you'll have produced another haircut that lives up to all claims of low maintenance, ignorable, healthy hair.

10.5 OTHER APPROACHES TO BULK-REMOVAL

When I work in my professional environment, I usually give a short, full cut by first cutting the upper two-thirds of the hair using the methods shown in the photos; for the bottom third, I use a clipper-over-comb cutting to get the hair tapered (page 178 has an abbreviated how-to). For me, with my experience, this is a quick and easy way to do it. But I find an **all** scissor and comb cutting, as shown on the cut-by-cut haircut, is needed in these situations:

● With little ones who are scared by the sound of the clippers.

● If I'm doing the cutting outdoors without access to electricity—a haircut outdoors is extra enjoyable for all involved.

You may eventually develop your skills to the point where you can use the faster clipper-over-comb way to taper the lower portions of the sides and back. But as a beginner, success is more easily achieved with the scissors-and-comb way to give short cuts.

In addition to choices of tools used, you may also choose a different cutting sequence for the short, full haircut.

1. After you have cut the top section, use the same stepping-out method around the sides and back that was recommended for the second-time-through part of the haircut. If you do it this way, your second-time cutting would require a vertical (diagonal around the bottom paths) HGH position around the sides and back.

2. Again, after the top section is cut in the usual manner, do the back section by stepping-out (horizontal HGH positioning). Then do the

* * *

Things are never the same between you when you have lied to someone.

Anonymous

A liar needs a good memory.

Quintilian

right and left sides with the vertical or diagonal HGH positioning.
For the second-time-through, use the vertical or diagonal position on
the back, and horizontal stepping-out cuts on the sides.
3. Occasionally, I do the edging first before any bulk-removal.

10.6 SHAPING OPTIONS WITH THE SHORT CUT

Short haircuts were my "bread and butter" throughout the 1960s; since
the late 1960s longer cuts have taken over, but shorter cuts still
make up a large percentage of my haircuts. Our survey of other ways to
give short haircuts begins with a look at recent haircutting history.

A. Short Cuts Aren't So Short

Prior to the 1970s, just about all edging around the ears and down the
sides of the neck was done as short and close to the natural hairline
as possible. In addition, the bottom neck hair was usually tapered
extra short.

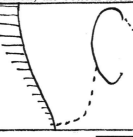

A "fresh-cut"
approach at
the neckline
has this
shape:

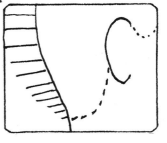

Short, full cuts are
left longer on the
bulk-removal, and
the line cut across
the bottom leaves
extra fullness.

An increasing number of folks
want the edgeline around the
ears, neckline,and sideburn
area left longer so the haircut
appears a few weeks old. The
idea is to cut the edge hair so
the cutting line is 1/2 - 3/4
inch away from the hairline.

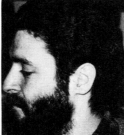

This "been worn awhile"
way of cutting is very
appropriate for those
who are changing from
a longer haircut to one
of these shorter cuts.

With this edgeline treatment, the extra neck hairs get a scissors-
over-comb cutting that leaves them about 1/2 inch long.

B. Short, Full Cut with a Longer Top

Short, full cuts can be given to virtually any head of hair with
excellent results. The major exception occurs with that rare person
who has a troublesome double cowlick that stands up if cut to a length
of 2 1/2 inches or shorter. If you encounter someone with a rooster
tail from twin cowlicks, leave the top 3 – 3 1/2 inches long so there
is enough extra length for the hair to bend into a lying position.
This extra-length cutting will need some tapering done to the hair on
pathways 4 and 5 on the top section. This tapering is done just on the
upper sides—not on the cutting around the upper back of the head.
With this extra length left on the top, you may have to cut off more
than the minimum amount when edge-cutting the bangs.

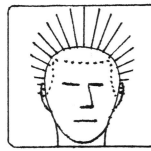
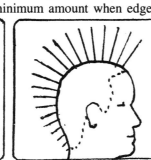
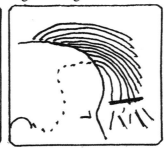
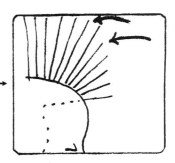

The arrows in the last illustration show the area that needs a little tapering after the bangs are cut. Take care of this with the second-time-through cutting.

Besides being a good length for the stand-on-end double cowlick, you'll find this is the length to leave straight hair if the top hair is worn toward the back despite its natural inclinations to lie toward the front: it takes extra length for it to bend.

C. The Extra Full, Short Cut

With this kind of shaping you achieve extra length and fullness around the sides and back, instead of on top as the previous option gave you.

1. **Bulk removal.** Give an equal-length cut to the whole head of hair. The best length would be 2 – 2 1/2 inches; however, it can be cut as short as 1 1/2 inches or as long as 3 inches, depending on texture or hairtype. If the hair around the bottom of the sides and back is shorter than the cutting length you have decided on, ignore those shorter hairs and go ahead and cut the rest of the hair to the desired length—those short ones get dealt with in the rest of the haircut. Taper the bottom neck hair using the stepping-out method while doing the bulk-removal.

2. **Edging.** Cut the bangs and temple region hair as you do on the equal-length cut. The edging around the the ears depends on hairgrain.

● Type 1 hairgrain. Cut in the edgeline the same way you did it on the short, full cut. However, to keep the extra fullness, do the edging away from the hairline—as close to the ear as possible.

● Type 2 hairgrain. Cut the edgeline in the ear area as you did for the equal-length cut. Here you want to have 1/2 – 1 inch of hair covering the top of the ear when the hair is combed straight down. When that hair is combed back so it lies in its preferred position, it lies above the ear, creating extra fullness.

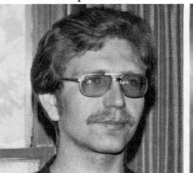 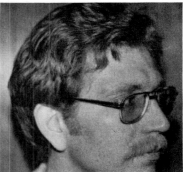

Combed down.   Combed back.

Do the edging down the sides of the neck as you did it for the equal-length cut. Because this cut has the neck hair tapered, your edgeline toward the bottom of the side of the neck conforms to that tapered cutting.

3. **A little tapering.** Besides tapering the neck hair somewhat, the hair that covers the ear will need some too if you cut off an inch or more while doing the edging there.

D. Finger Cut

Because my hair is as fine as frog's hair, plus a forehead that seems to grow every year, and I have the short-growing hair problem around the lower sides, this is my haircut. (With all these hair conditions, I don't have much choice.) On this cut you are actually giving an equal-length cut, except that here there is no space between the scalp and the holding fingers—they lie flat on the scalp. Cutting off all the hair that protrudes above the holding fingers leaves the hair 3/4 – 1 inch long all over. Follow the same sequence of cuts used on the equal-length cut. This is the easiest of the short cuts to give—it's in this part of the chapter because its short length is not adaptable to many heads of hair.

This cut works especially well with soft, baby-fine, straight or wavy hair—the coarser varieties will stand on end if cut this short. When it comes to curly or kinky hair, it doesn't make any difference if the hair is baby-fine or as coarse as #14 wire: it lies in closely spaced waves or stands out in smoothly cut curls—even with the skinniest of holding fingers.

With the exception of the lower temple region, do all the edging as you did it for the short, full cut. The lower temple, because of the equal-length bulk-removal, needs to be cut with the edgeline equal distance from the hairline.

If past experience is a good predictor of tomorrow's haircuts, we will see a wide variety of hair-dos come and go—the haircutting skills you've learned should leave you well-equipped to handle anything that comes along. Even though new ways of wearing hair are bound to appear, the haircuts that remain popular have always been the ones with the characteristics of practicality and simplicity. This being the case, it's quite likely that shingles-on-a-roof cutting and these three basic ways of doing it will be going strong as long as hair is cut!

The last chapter presents miscellaneous bits of haircutting knowledge that didn't seem to fit into any of the earlier chapters.

* * *

Freedom rings where opinions clash.   Anonymous
There are two ways to slide easily through life; to believe everything or to doubt everything; both ways save us from thinking.   A. Korzybski
Justifying a fault doubles it.   Anonymous
If fifty-million people say a foolish thing, it is still a foolish thing.   Anatole France
People should think things out fresh and not just accept conventional terms and the conventional way of doing things.   Buckminster Fuller
Every society honors its live conformists and its dead troublemakers.
                    Migno McLaughlin
We must have courage to bet on our ideas, to take the calculated risk, and to act. Everday living requires courage if life is to be effective and bring happiness.   Maxwell Maltz
The great law of culture: Let each become all that he was created capable of being.   Thomas Carlyle
That man is a success who has lived well, laughed often and loved much; who has gained the respect of intelligent men and the love of children; who has filled his niche and accomplished his task; who leaves the world better than he found it, whether by an improved poppy, a perfect poem or a rescued soul; who never lacked appreciation of earth's beauty or failed to express it; who looked for the best in others and gave the best he had.   Robert Louis Stevenson
It is the chiefest point of happiness that a man is willing to be what he is.   Desiderius Erasmus
To own a bit of ground, to scratch it with a hoe, to plant seeds, and watch the renewal of life—this is the commonest delight of the race, the most satisfying thing a man can do.   Charles Dudley Warner
Man—despite his artistic pretensions, his sophistication, and his many accomplishments—owes his existence to a six-inch layer of topsoil and the fact that it rains.   Anonymous
The real purpose of books is to trap the mind into doing its own thinking.   Christopher Morley

11 SNIPS AND TIPS

11.1 CUTTING CHILDREN'S HAIR

Little people need special handling to keep their locks in good shape.

A. **Their Hair and its Needs**
Children's hair almost always starts out on the finer side and slowly
gets coarser until they reach puberty—this has consequences for you:
1. **Frequent haircutting**. The fine hair of childhood is inevitably
weaker hair that is much more prone to damage. Damaged hair = tangled
hair = painful hair whenever it's groomed or shampooed = hair that
usually doesn't get the kind of haircare it needs. Don't wait until
the hair and its care becomes a painful drudgery; instead, set a
regular haircutting schedule of once every four to six weeks. With the
benefits that come from your cutting efforts, this will be remembered
as a very positive time for the child and you. When you give the
haircuts taught in this book, just about all the ends are cut off—the
pain-causing culprits are on the floor instead of on the head.
2. **Delicate hair**. Because finer hair is most affected by the many
ways it can be damaged, the dos and don'ts **should** be closely
followed. Pain-free hair is possible and it's every child's **right.**
3. **Cut children's hair on the shorter side**. As chapter 7 pointed
out, if a head of fine hair is to hold a good shape all the time—with
the recommended shampoo and towel-dry approach to haircare—it has to
be cut shorter than larger diameter hair. Cutting that limp, messy
prone hair shorter gives it some body and fullness and keeps it lying
well no matter what the active child's day may bring. The shorter
lengths also are much less likely to tangle and snarl. As a child
matures, be aware of and accommodate your cutting to the hair's more
coarse texture.

B. **Safety Considerations**
Usually a 3 – 4 year old child is able to sit still and be helpful—
but I've worked on one-year-olds who sat better than some adults (?)
do. If you have a cooperative youngster, you won't have to do anything
special. Those movers and shakers are a different story: they'll need
out-of-the-ordinary tactics to do the job **safely** and **quickly**.
1. **Kinds of haircuts to give**. Because of sudden movements and the

possibility of injury from the points of the scissors, always limit yourself to the equal-length or long, layered cuts. During the short, full cut, the scissors operate close to the skin; the longer haircuts have the cutting occur at least 1 – 2 inches farther away from the skin—an important margin of safety to have on your side. In addition, the extra preciseness of the short, full cut makes it a long, drawn-out experience, and more than likely a disaster in terms of smooth, even cutting if you have a wiggler.

2. **Time factor**. You want to get done as quickly as possible when you work on a little one who can't sit still. You won't wear the child down, but they'll wear you out. Forgo the second-time-through cutting and accept the less even cutting results—everyone is better off.

3. **An extra shortcut**. One good way to speed up the haircutting process and avoid any close contact of blades with the skin is to forget the edge-cutting. The bulk-removal makes the edgeline hair conform to the hairline, so very little cutting needs to be done to those edge hairs. Better safe than sorry, even if those edge hairs aren't cut as well as possible.

C. Ways to Get Maximum Cooperation

1. **Get the child used to it**. Spend some time for a few days before the haircut, familiarizing the child with the spray bottle, combing through the hair, and holding the hair out from the scalp. You don't want any surprises on haircut day.

2. **Timing can be crucial**. From my experience I've found it's easiest to cut children's hair right after they wake up from a nap: they always seem to be in a pleasant, fuzzy state that minimizes nervous energies and crankiness.

3. **Before the nap**. To avoid starting the haircut session with any pain, shampoo, dry, and thoroughly brush out the child's hair.

4. **Someone to help**. Your helper has a few important functions:

● Keep the child's attention. Little ones are usually very curious about that clicking sound they hear as you're snipping away. They turn their head this way and that to see what is going on—not very conducive to being stationary. Use whatever means possible (toys, a key chain, conversation) to keep their mind off what you're doing.

● Provide your helper with a hair duster, folded napkin, or wash cloth to keep those ticklish cut-hairs off the child's face and neck.

● A lap for a chair. It is hard for a little child to sit alone on a chair or stool—in a short time their back aches and they move around in an effort to get comfortable. Have your helper sit on a chair with the child seated on the helper's knees. Face the child toward the helper and you will have plenty of working room. You might be better off not to use a haircloth on children: some don't like to have their hands and arms covered up. Your helper can also help out by gently holding the child's head in a convenient position for you.

● Extra help. If it doesn't get too crowded, you may want two helpers: one is the holder and the other is the distractor who also keeps the hair off the child's sensitive skin.

5. **Be positive**. Keep a pleasant, soft voice to encourage the child's helpfulness. Positive reinforcement always works best.

11.2 BEARD TRIMMING

A. Facial Hair Options

The last fifteen years has brought a major change in the way men deal

with their face hair. In the 1950s a moustache was rare, a beard much
rarer. Today a majority (or close to it) of men wear some form of
facial hair. Many times a man will go through these growing stages
before he is ready for full hairgrowth on the face.

1. **Mustache.**

Step one is to grow some hair
on the upper lip. This growth
may go just to the corners
of the mouth or it may grow
down a ways:

2. **The goatee appears.**

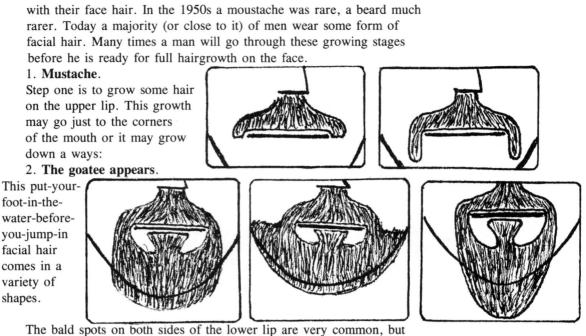

This put-your-
foot-in-the-
water-before-
you-jump-in
facial hair
comes in a
variety of
shapes.

The bald spots on both sides of the lower lip are very common, but
many men have solid hairgrowth below the lower lip.

3. **Then comes the beard.** The beard, like the goatee, can be cut
and/or shaved into many different shapes. The following two approaches
are the most common: they both need a fairly short (1/2 – 1 inch)
equal-length cutting all over the growing area—the difference between
the two depends on whether you choose to shave part of the face.

● Partial shaving. Shave the upper and/or lower portions of the beard.
Whichever way it's done, you normally shave in the edgeline so that it
is parallel to the jawline (the dotted line).

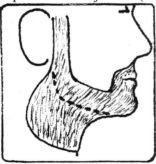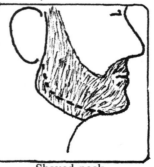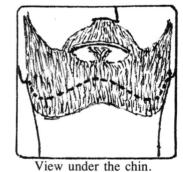

Shaved cheek area.   Shaved neck.   View under the chin.

I think the main advantage of a beard is lost if some portion of it
has to be shaved—perhaps that's why this next beard is so popular.

● The emancipated shaver. The most low-maintenance beard is the kind
that gets an equal-length cut all over once every 2 – 6 weeks.

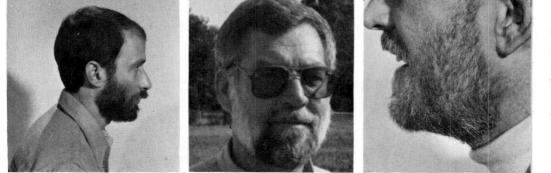

The majority of
the beards I
see (and the
beard trimming
I do) is of
this type.

B. **How to Trim the Beard: The Scissors-Over-Comb Way to Cut**
Your cutting goal when you trim a partially shaved beard or no-shave
beard is a fairly short equal-length cut. In the barbershop I usually
use a clipper-over-comb method of cutting. Sometimes I use the clipper
with a spacer guide—an old time "butch" haircut for the whiskers.

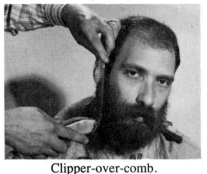
Clipper-over-comb.

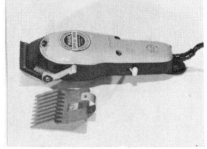
Tools for a "butch".

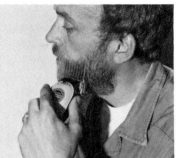
Using clipper and spacer.

The same equal-length cutting results can be achieved by the scissors-
over-comb cutting technique—it just takes longer. This cutting method
has some new ways to use hands and tools. In a nutshell, you keep the
comb flat and equal distance from the skin as it travels through the
beard. The scissors follow along, cutting the hair that protrudes from
the comb. Here are the specifics of this way of cutting:

1. **Comb handling**.

● Direct the comb through the hair, going against or sideways to the
beard grain. The beard hair builds up at the backbar of the comb, and
you cut just in front of the backbar. This build-up has the hair
standing straight out from the skin for the cutting—just as the HGH
holds the hair out from the head during bulk-cutting. Here the comb is
the spacer tool instead of your hand.

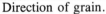
Direction of grain.

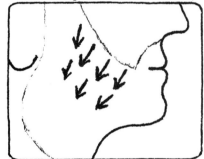
Comb goes this way.

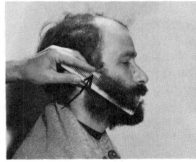
Or this way.

● Most important, you must maintain your comb at a **consistent**
distance from the skin as it travels through the hair. The scissors
cut only those hairs that protrude above the comb, so you need to pay
close attention to the comb's distance from the skin. This is a
bit more difficult when the comb passes over the curved areas of the
jaw and chin—just go slowly and carefully manipulate the comb.

● Use the guide-hair aid
from the paths you cut.
The comb goes through the
hair in paths that are
alongside of paths
that have just been cut.
The ends of the
guide-hair appear at
backbar, toward the
comb's tip or the handle.

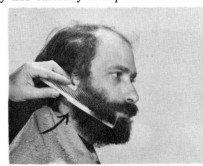

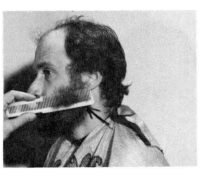

As usual, don't shorten any of the guide hairs—just use them so the uncut hairs get cut to the same length. Use those helping hairs, but focus your primary attention on the comb's distance from the skin.

● The comb's thickness. The average comb is about 1/4 inch thick. If you hold the comb 1/4 inch away from the skin, you end up with a 1/2 inch beard length.

● Unsnagging the comb. When the comb travels against or sideways to the grain, it's easily snagged—especially when you start out through the hair. To get moving again, pivot the comb's backbar away from the skin 1/2 inch.

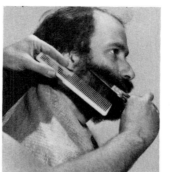 Slip the closed scissors under the comb, up to the snagged hairs. Remove the comb.

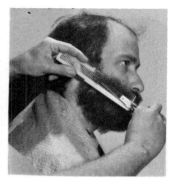 Reinsert comb under scissors. Reposition scissors at the backbar, and you're ready to move on.

2. Scissors handling.

As the photos in this section show, the comb is the "director": it sets up the hair and determines how much will be cut. The scissors are in a secondary role of just cutting the hair that the comb produces.

● Remember, cut a little in front of the comb's backbar.

● Make a cut for each 1/2 inch (or less) of the comb's travel through the hair.

● You open and then close the blades all the way while cutting. As you're doing this, you insure a smoother, more even cutting if you open the blades fairly wide and cut with more of the center part of the blades. Short cuts at the points of the blades usually produces an uneven cutting.

● You're better able to keep the scissors snipping just in front of the backbar when you—as much as possible—do your cutting by moving the thumb blade: keep the fingers blade as stationary as you can.

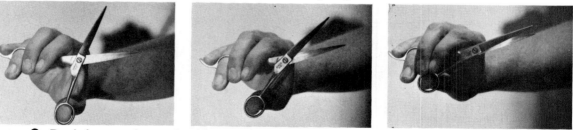

● Don't lean on the comb with your scissors as you cut. Hold the cutters so they lightly touch or are about 1/8 inch from the comb.

3. Practice.

You need to practice the scissors-over-comb method before you are clicking along without effort. Use the same practice I used in barber school: the rookie students would stand around a pole in the center of the school's shop area, clicking away with comb and scissors at imaginery hair "growing" from the pole. A goofy sight, but it got both hands working together. You can do your practice on a door jam. For more realism, find a beard wearer who doesn't really care how short his beard is cut. If you botch things up, it won't matter if the smooth-off cutting leaves the beard as short as 1/4 – 3/8 inch (the shortest it can be cut when you add the comb's thickness).

C. Tapering the Beard

An equal-length cutting is the simplest and best way to trim beards. However, many men have a hairgrain clash in the lower neck area that makes the beard stand on end. A little tapering keeps this area in good shape.

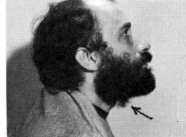

The tapering is done to the hair **above** those stand out hairs. But first you deal with the hair at the clash point and the hair below it.

1. Insert the comb a little above the stand out hairs.

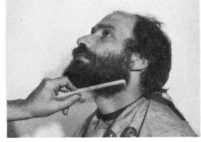

Comb downward while holding the comb flat against the skin. Cut the hair as short as possible (about 1/4 inch). It takes several paths to get all the lower hair cut.

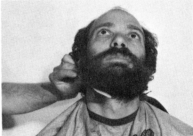

2. Start tapering the hair (above the clash point) where your short cutting on the lower neck began. Insert the comb into the hair, flat against the skin.

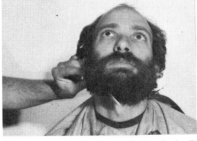

Then pivot the teeth of the comb out and away from the skin, while you maintain skin contact with the backbar:

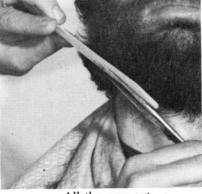

Move the comb through the hair **following** the direction the teeth point toward. The backbar loses contact with the skin as soon as the comb begins its trip through the hair: you have to be sure the comb travels in the same direction you establish in the beginning position.

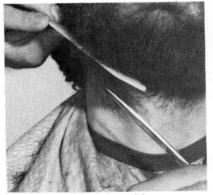

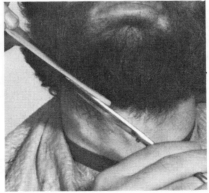

Beginning position.   Halfway out.   All the way out.

(Hair was being cut during the shooting of these photos—the timing was just a little off as the shutter snapped and the scissors closed.)

As with the short cutting on the lower neck hair, it takes several paths to get all of the upper neck hair tapered. Be sure to use that guide-hair after the first path.

How far the teeth are pointed away from the skin when you first position the comb determines how gradual or abrupt the tapering is. If you pivot the teeth only 1/4 inch away from the skin, you'll have a longer, more gradual taper; 1/2 inch or more from the skin makes the taper fairly abrupt.

This way to taper hair can also be used around the bottom of a short, full cut or in place of the tapering methods shown for the equal-length cut's neck hair. Before using this cutting method on haircuts, you should stay with beard trimming until you have enough success to feel comfortable with it.

D. Miscellaneous Beard Tips

1. **Length**. The question of beard length is a matter of personal preference; however, most prefer their beard trimmed so it has less fullness than their haircut. To achieve this, curlier and coarse, wiry beards would be cut shorter than the straighter, finer varieties that lie down—most of my beard trims are in the 3/8 – 3/4 inch range. If you leave the whiskers longer than 1 inch, you could do the cutting with the same holding-guide-hand methods as used for haircutting.

2. **Avoid harsh soap**. While beard hair tends to be more coarse and less prone to damage, it can end up very tangly/snarly when bar soap is used to wash it. This problem is simple to avoid: just use the same low pH shampoo you use on those locks—shampooing them together saves time and effort. (That low pH cleanser is easy on the skin too.)

3. **The itchy grow-out**. When a clean-shaven man starts to grow a beard, he can expect about 1 – 2 weeks of the scratchy itchies. The reason for this is not known, but it is a rare fellow who isn't affected by this distracting condition. You can minimize the problem by thoroughly washing the growing out stubble several times a day. Other than this, all you can do is **endure**, with the sure knowledge that it will soon be over. (It doesn't return when the beard is trimmed short, but it does if the beard is shaved off and regrown.)

11.3 HAIRCUTTING AROUND THE WORLD

While most of my haircutting has been to American Caucasians, being a barber in the U.S.A. has allowed me to give haircuts to people from all corners of the world and to all the major races. There are many exceptions to the generalizations I make here, but I'm confident these statements are a fairly accurate picture of the wide world of hair.

A. Southeast Asians and Native Americans

With rare exception, these people have black or graying hair and it's almost always straight with a coarser texture. 80 – 90 percent have a Type 1 hairgrain, and they don't experience baldness as much as Caucasians. All three basic haircuts work well. However, you should plan on giving the longer versions with this kind of coarse hair.

* * *

There is no more evil thing in this world than race prejudice . . . It justifies and holds together more baseness, cruelty, and abomination than any other sort of error in the world.   H. G. Wells

Racism is man's greatest threat to man—the maximum of hatred for a minimum of reason.   Abraham Joshua Heschel

B. **Blacks**

Black people's hair ranges from curly to extra kinky. Normally the texture is coarse and they tend to have many hairs per square inch. Blacks come second (after Caucasians) in being affected by baldness.

The haircuts you have learned here are all very adaptable to this kind of hair. The equal-length cut, called the Afro or Fro, is the most popular of the three. Curly and kinky hair is easier to handle when using a large, heavy duty comb. If the hair is extra hard to comb through, give it a hot oil treatment before the haircut (see page 35).

Professionals who have a lot of experience cutting Blacks' hair usually use the free-hand clipper-cutting method or the scissors-over-comb technique. Both are faster and easier ways to cut, but both—especially clipper-cutting—require much experience and skill.

C. **Caucasians**

There is a fairly distinct difference between the hair qualities of Caucasians, depending on whether they come from northern Europe, or the Mediterranean, Middle East, and North Africa.

1. **Northerners**.
● Redheads and brunets abound, but close to a majority have blond hair—from darker blond to the nearly-white blond.
● Hair texture is on the finer side, and they usually have straight or slightly wavy hair.
● With many exceptions, they usually have a Type 1 hairgrain.
● Instead of total baldness, they tend to have a thinned-out hairloss.

2. **Folks around the Mediterranean**.
● Brunet and especially black hair is the rule here.
● Hair texture is medium to coarse, and they usually have wavy or curly hair—the farther south you go, the curlier it gets.
● Type 2 hairgrain on just about everyone.
● Hairloss tends to be complete, especially on the eastern and southern sides of the Mediterranean. On the western side, the Spanish and Portugese are well known for hanging onto their hair.

D. **Other groups**.

1. People from the subcontinent of India have hair similar to those who live around the Mediterranean. However, curly hair is not so common, and they are not affected as much by baldness.
2. Canadians, for the most part, have the northern hair qualities of their English heritage, or the southern qualities of their French ancestors, or the characteristics of Native Americans.
3. Our Hispanic neighbors to the south have dark hair that ranges from straight to kinky depending on ancestry: Native American, Spanish and Portugese, and Black. Type 2 hairgrain prevails except for Native Americans, and the texture is on the coarser side. Baldness is not as common as it is for those in the more northern climes.

11.4 FOUR SEASONS HAIRCUTTING

This is a common sense, ever changing way of cutting and wearing the hair that results from living in an always changing weather environment. In Minnesota, U.S.A., the temperatures range from 95 – 100 hot humid degrees, to −80 or −90 degrees (when you figure the wind

* * *

If a man does not keep pace with his companions, perhaps it is because he hears a different drummer.
                                                                    Henry David Thoreau

chill factor). With this wide-ranging temperature, hair can be an ally
or an enemy, depending on how long or short it is. The weather-wise
Minnesotan changes their type of haircut according to the temperature
changes. A typical cutting cycle goes like this:

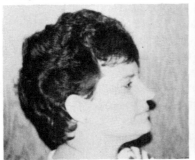

June: short, full
(top is extra full).

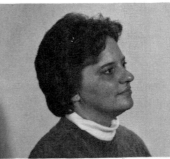

September: short
equal-length.

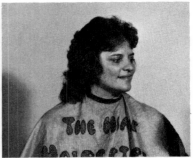

December: long, layered
(umbrella version).

March: long
equal-length.

This practical-minded approach makes burdensome
hair into a good thing to have around. Success
with this kind of haircutting scheme depends on
the kind of hair you have to work with, but you
will find a majority of your haircuttees can
enjoy this haircut flexibility. The only kinds
of hair that won't fit into this weather
cutting routine are very fine straight hair, or
problem hair that limits what can be done.

11.5 YOUR HAIRCUTTING RESULTS WILL SURPRISE YOU

Cutting hair definitely is a funny business. Many times, after giving
my best cutting effort while following the length and shaping rules
laid out in chapter 7, I've found my results on hair with problems has
left me feeling disappointed. No, the hair didn't lie as well as I
hoped; but, more times than not, that person came back for a second
haircut, telling me their first haircut was the best they had ever
received. These people have lived a long time with their problem hair
and have put up with a long string of poor haircuts along the way. I
always try hard, and the hair knowledge I've built up over the years
(while it may not make a masterpiece out of a difficult head of hair)
does maximize the hair's ability to lie well and look good. The folks
with problem hair usually end up being my best customers.

Give the hair you're working on your best guess and best effort:
more times than not you will do a very good job, probably a whole lot
better than you give yourself credit for.

It is a funny business and it's fun too!

11.6 HAIRTYPE ISN'T ALWAYS WHAT IT APPEARS TO BE

Depending on length and haircare, hair takes on different appearances.
You may think you have a particular type of hair to work on, but in
fact, it is something quite different.

A. The Many Faces of Wavy Hair
● Cut wavy hair short enough (1 – 2 inches) and it takes on the

appearance of straight hair that has a lot of body and fullness. This
first photo shows a 2 inch equal-length cut.

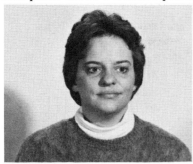

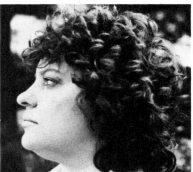

● When wavy hair gets long
enough (2 – 3 inches) it
regains its waviness. Grow
the hair longer (3 – 5
inches) and it takes on a
curly appearance. This
photo was taken about 4
months after the one on
the left—no haircuts
during that time.

● When you grow wavy hair to a length of 10 – 12 inches or more, the
weight plus the force of gravity pulls it straight, especially around
the upper 2/3 of the hair.

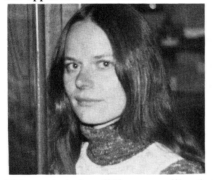

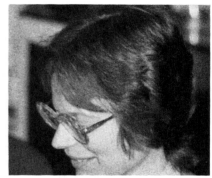

When you give hair
like this a long,
layered cut, (in
this case it got
the umbrella
version,) some
waviness returns
because the extra
weight is gone.

If Long hair is a little wavy, like that shown in the photo on the
left, it shows its waviness down around the bottom—there isn't any
weight pulling on the hair down there.

B. Straight Hair that Looks Wavy, Even a Little Curly

If finer textured straight hair, with a Type 2 hairgrain, is grown
long enough, the hair around the lower sides and back appears wavy or
curly. This isn't because the hair has changed its hairtype, it's due
to weight and gravity causing the hair to bend downward—a direction
contrary to the hair's druthers. In this case, you're seeing flippy
hair: it may appear curly, but when that excess length and weight are
cut off, the hair returns to its natural way of lying and the false
waves or curls are gone.

Flippiness results when fine,
straight hair with a Type 2
grain is grown to a length
of 4 – 6 inches. The same
hair at 2 – 3 inches long
often flips forward at the
lower temple region. Cut it
shorter and it will
feather-back naturally.

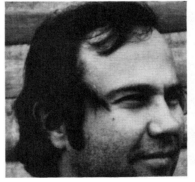

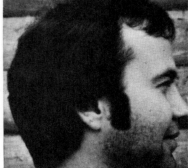

C. Curly Hair that Looks Wavy

If curly hair is cut to a length of 1 inch or less, it usually lies
into waves. Let it grow another 1/2 inch and it curls again.

D. Haircare's Impact

As if there wasn't enough to deal with in solving this hairtype puzzle, now we add how the hair is cared for. How the hair is dried and how often it is shampooed will affect the hair's true nature.

● If you don't shampoo often enough, your natural oil accumulation causes the hairs to cling together. This condition makes straight hair appear wavy, wavy hair gets curly, and curly hair gets curlier (the same is true for the use of too much hairdressing). Infrequent shampooing means the hair also gets kinked up and bent from being slept on, giving a curlier appearance.

● When wavy hair is allowed to dry naturally, with towel-drying plus air-drying, or just air-drying, the wet hairs cling to their neighbors and wavy hair becomes curly, straight hair gets a little wavy, and so on. If the hair is drummed-dry, it lies much straighter.

11.7 TRIMMING BANGS

You already know how to trim the bangs for the different haircuts; here you learn how to cut bangs when that's the only cutting to be done. How you trim the bangs depends largely on how the hair has been cut in the past, and how much length is desired for the rest of the hair—other than the bangs.

A. Growing Out the Three Haircuts
When any of our three haircuts are grown out, they eventually need some trimming to permit 20/20 vision. Whether your cutting is confined to just the bangs, or if it also includes the temple region hair, depends on **how much** the hair is to be grown out.

1. If you're just being a bit lazy, and only want to remove a little vision-obscuring hair (instead of giving a complete haircut), all the hair that frames the face should be cut. This is necessary, especially on straighter hair, because temple hair falls forward into the corners of the eyes if it's left too long. The same edging methods are used on this trimming as used when you gave the haircut.

2. If the side hair is to grow out for a time, but the bangs need some trimming—you have to take care to avoid cutting any of the side hair.

This is easily done by combing the side hair down and toward the back of the head. Comb the bangs straight forward onto the forehead. Trim the bangs to the desired length; but they are usually left long enough to reach the part of the temple hairline that protrudes furthest toward the face.

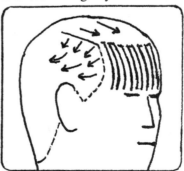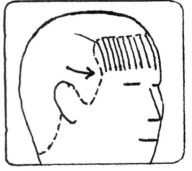

B. Trimming Bangs on Perimeter-Cut Hair
If you are working on a longer head of hair that has only received perimeter cuts in the past, your trim methods change a little, depending on **how much** of the hair's perimeter has been cut before.

1. **Tree shape**. If the hair's perimeter has been cut into a tree shape like it was done on a long, layered cut, you only need to repeat

* * *

If God had meant for us to have pay toilets, we would have been born with correct change.   Anonymous

Undermine the entire structure of society by leaving the pay toilet door ajar so the next person can get in free.   Taylor Mead the same edge-cutting you're familiar with (see pages 142 – 145).

2. **Bottom only**. Long hair that has only received perimeter cutting around the bottom of the sides and back will need some unusual parting of the hair before the bangs can be cut. Here you will be cutting bangs where there weren't any before. Creating bangs and where you part the hair depend on the **kind** of hair you have to work with. These are the two basic ways to do it:

● **The "V" part**. Use this part with a Type 1 hairgrain that has the top hair growing forward, or a Type 2 hairgrain with a natural part at (or near) the center of the top of the head. You make a **double** part from the corners of the front hairline to a point back (usually 1 1/2 – 2 inches) from the center of the front hairline, thus forming a "V".

The farther back the two parts meet, the heavier (more hair) the bangs will be. If the two parts meet close to the front hairline, the bangs have a wispy appearance.

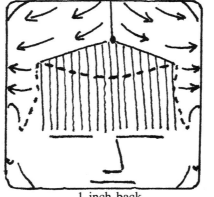

1 inch back.

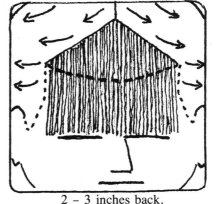

2 – 3 inches back.

After you part the hair, first pin back the side hair and the long top hair behind the parting with barettes or bobby pins. Comb the hair within the "V" onto the forehead and trim. If the bangs are to lie on the forehead, ignore the shape of the top front hairline as you cut the bangs straight across—use the pull-and-cut followed by the finger-bracing-the-scissors method for stragglers. If you want the bangs to lie somewhat downward and then back toward the upper side hair, trim the bangs so they are equal distance from the underlying hairline and leave them with an extra 1 – 2 inches of length—use the modified-bulk-removal edging method.

● **A side part**. When the top front hair wants to lie naturally toward one side or the other (with either Type 1 or Type 2 hairgrain), the parting procedure for the bangs is changed. After determining which side the hair is to be parted on (see pages 87 through 89), comb the long top hair to the side.

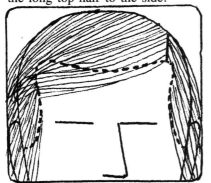

Then make a part that starts 1 – 2 inches behind the hairline on the part side, and goes over to the opposite corner at the hairline.

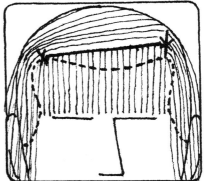

Again, pin the top and side hair out of your way. Trim the bangs as you did for "V" parting or use the modified-bulk-removal method and follow the shape of the hairline. This type of bangs will swoop-off to the side with the rest of the top hair, so you need to do the cutting

1 – 2 inches longer than what you want for the final lying position.

The how-to descriptions for creating bangs also work for trimming existing bangs that are too long.

C. Variations

1. **The edge line**. Bangs can be cut: straight across, conforming to the shape of the forehead's hairline, or with curved corners. The first two options don't need any more explanation; the third one does.

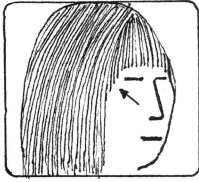

Pin the side and top hair back. Pinch the bangs into a single strand and make one cut at the bridge of the nose (or higher). Follow up with a finger-bracing-the-scissors method to trim any stragglers.

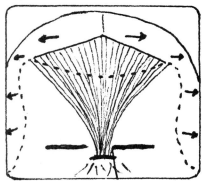

2. **Soften the bottom of the bangs**. If you want the bangs less heavy at the bottom, you can layer them a little. Cutting off 1/4 inch or less with the HGH held in these approximate positions will do the trick. Each position shown is preceded by a comb-out.

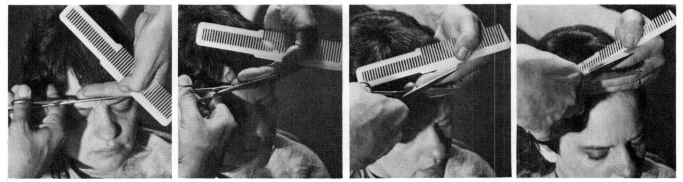

11.8 CUTTING YOUR OWN HAIR

I bought some real estate from an elderly minister some years back. As we were chatting while the papers were being drawn up, he told me haircutters and bartenders had the biggest opportunity to do some good for their fellow humans. According to his thinking, we had the most time to spend in a one-on-one personal service that had the potential to be very positive. Maybe pouring alcohol for people can be helpful, but there is no doubt in my mind that helping someone with their hair needs can, indeed, be a very positive thing to do for others. Because of this view, I can't get enthusiastic about the do-it-to-yourself approach: there is a world full of people who would be more than happy to learn this skill—share the book so you can exchange cutting efforts, and enjoy the social benefits.

Besides social considerations, cutting your own hair is a tough task. Difficult for all who attempt it, most find it an awkward process that takes too much effort for results that usually disappoint. There are people who cut their own and do a good job—I wonder how many disasterous cuttings they had to wear before they perfected their skills?

* * *

The measure of life is not duration, but rather its donation.   Anon.

The lonely way of cutting needs a mirror, and for the cutting around the back, two mirrors. I feel somewhat awkward when I look in the mirror to trim the bottom of my mustache—to have to use two mirrors would really discombobulate me.

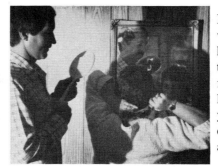

It looks like a good way to cut the holding fingers. Get together with a friend who wants to learn this skill— you'll make life easier on yourself and your fingers.

Trimming your beard is quite easy if you use a clipper with the spacer attachment. The scissors-over-comb method is a possibility, but like giving yourself a haircut, it is a slow awkward process.

11.9 HAIRCUTTER AS A MERCHANT OF CHANGE

Here we all are, living in a universe of change. It goes on all the time in the heavens above and in the physical and social environment that surrounds us. Add to this a physical self that is in a constant state of change from our first day to our last, and it's obvious that change is the most natural thing going on.

As a haircutter you fit into this ever-changing world because you **create change**. Everytime you close the scissors on a handful of hairs, change happens. The majority of your haircuts will be trims: you just cut off the hair that has grown out since the last haircut— the change made here is not significant. On many of the first-time haircuts you give, you'll make notable changes by cutting the hair quite a bit shorter or by giving it a different shape. You need to remember that people react differently to change—awareness of this can make all difference between successful and discouraging results.

A. How People Handle the Change a Haircut Brings: Four Categories

There are good reasons why people are referred to as individuals. As such, I'm always leery of attempts to categorize people, yet my experience teaches me these four categories are fairly accurate descriptions of most people. At the risk of over-simplifying, this information is offered in the hope it helps you avoid people pitfalls.

1. **The positive type**. Given a good haircut that is easy to care for, these folks are happy about the change that has happened to their hair. Typically, these people are self-assured enough to handle any amount of change when it proves to be a better way. From 1/4 – 1/3 of my first-timers are in this category.

2. **The neutral type**. About 1/5 of the population could care less about the change a different haircut brings—all they want is to get it off. These are the functional-minded ones who don't want to see the mirror—they just appreciate being rid of a burden. (Don't be shocked when later they compliment you on your precision cutting skills.)

3. **The change-is-hard people**. Nearly a majority of your first-timers will be folks whose initial reaction to what has happened to their changed hair is something less than positive. They leave you feeling defeated after your best efforts have produced a haircut you know is well done. The thing to keep in mind is **give them time.** The undeniable benefits of this kind of haircutting and haircare soon become obvious to them. In addition, these folks do listen to and are

* * *

It's the most unhappy people who most fear change. Mignon McLaughlin affected by the compliments they will get on their new haircut. Most, if not all, of us have some insecurity with change, but in this case a better way proves itself in a short time—soon the insecurities are forgotten and your efforts are appreciated.

4. **The white-knuckle, no-change folks**. You could spend an hour or two giving someone the best haircut that person has ever had and still have an unhappy—maybe even slightly hostile—haircuttee on your hands. I'm referring to a minority of people who have a knee-jerk way of reacting to any kind of change—it is always **NO**! Even with compliments and the easy care advantages being evident, the uptight ones won't be able to accept what has happened to their hair—no matter how much time you give them. I am very thankful these people are a small percentage of the haircuttee population, otherwise cutting hair would be one of the worst ways of spending time and efforts. This small minority is even smaller as far as you're concerned: their hair is **so important** to them, few would trust their haircut needs to a home haircutter.

B. Avoiding People Problems

To go from a somewhat unsure, perhaps nervous beginner to a veteran haircutter who enjoys the craft, you need to choose the **right** folks for your early haircuts. Maximize your chances for success by avoiding the people in categories 3 and 4, and work your rookie status off on the easy-to-get-along-with folks in 1 and 2. When experience has built your confidence and your hands and tools are clicking along, then you'll be in good shape to handle the more difficult folks.

C. Gradual Change

Most people have a hard time with a major change in the way their hair is cut (even, sometimes, if they tell you that is what they want). Unless you are dealing with a fairly rare person, you should minimize the change trauma by gradually cutting the hair shorter. Let's say you are going to give a haircut to someone with the kind of long hair that has only had perimeter cuts in the past. The first haircut should be a long, layered cut, later a fairly long equal-length cut, then maybe a shorter equal-length, and then, if desired, one of the short cuts.

11.10 CLIPPER-OVER-COMB CUTTING

This subject, plus detailed how-to for different clipper haircuts, could be my next book or pamphlet-length writing project. Here I'll explain, in brief, the general rules for clipper-over-comb cutting.

The tools to use are the same long-toothed comb used for scissors cutting, and any good-cutting clipper—the adjustable blade clipper shown on page 167 is excellent.

This method of cutting can be used to taper the lower sides and back hair on a short haircut (chapter 10, sections 2-B and 5), and for tapering the neck area of beards (see pages 167 to 169 for a little review). The how-to for this cutting has a number of similarities to the cutting methods you've already learned, and a couple of changes:

1. **Dry hair**. This cutting has to be done with the hair dry because wet hair clumps together and does not feed well into the blades.

2. **The comb's function**. The hair must stand straight out from the scalp while being cut—as it was for bulk-cutting. Like scissors-over-cutting (page 167), the comb holds the hair out instead of the HGH.

3. **Cutting direction**. When using the finger-bracing method, the

scissors has to travel against or sideways to the direction of the grain—the same is true for this cutting. Once the comb is positioned with the hair to be cut held out from the scalp, the clippers travel over the comb—lightly scraping the side of the comb's teeth—in a direction that is against (or at least sideways to) the hairgrain.

4. **Comb's position**. As it was when tapering with the scissors-over-comb method, the comb's teeth point away from the skin—how much it points away is what determines how gradual or abrupt the taper is.

5. **The cutting**. Position the comb's backbar at the hairline (and parallel to it), pivot the teeth away from the skin for 1/2 – 3/4 inch and cut the hair protruding from the comb. For example, if you are doing the bottom neck hair, the comb is positioned horizontally and the clipper also travels horizontally—to the left or right.

6. **Keep cutting until you're out of the hair**. As with scissors-over-comb cutting, you keep cutting until the comb is out of the hair. If a second cut is to be made higher up into the hair, position the comb—with the same angle away from the scalp—above the first cutting (now the backbar won't be in contact with the skin). Then hold the comb stationary as you make the next cutting across the comb.

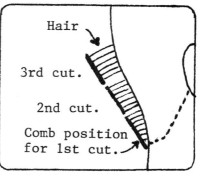

7. **Your focus**. Like scissors-over-comb cutting, the comb is the primary tool because it determines how much hair is cut off; the clippers are in a secondary role of only cutting off the hair that protrudes from the comb. Pay close attention to the positioning of the comb, and don't lean heavily on the comb with the clippers.

8. **Guide-hair**. As it was with scissors-over-comb cutting, do your cutting beside an already-cut area so you can have some of that cut hair at the tip of the comb or toward the handle—once the comb is positioned for cutting. If you are making a second cut, higher up into the hair, you should also have guide-hair at the backbar of the comb. Look closely to avoid cutting any guide-hair.

11.11 DEALING WITH PERMANENT HAIRLOSS

There are a wide variety of ways to deal with permanent hairloss: the possibilities range from the surgeon's scalpel to simple acceptance. This first option is the most expensive and least popular.

A. Hair Transplants
This is the Robin Hood approach where you take from the rich and give to the poor. In this procedure, an M.D. takes a "plug" of several growing hairs from the side or back of the head and embeds it in the meager top. A number of these plugs, surgically transplanted, are an effective, long lasting but not permanent solution to hairloss. The main drawbacks are the high cost and pain. I've known several fellows who had this done: each complained about the fee and headaches they endured during the time it took to get some hair growing again.

B. Hairpiece
I don't know what got into me back in 1972—I suppose a burst of vanity/insecurity—when I bought a custom-made hairpiece for my easily sunburned dome. It took about a week before I chucked it and

accepted reality. From first-hand experience, I know a rug is:
- Expensive. At least $400 – $500 for a better quality version, and upwards of $10 a month for cleaning supplies and tape or glue.
- Uncomfortable. It is hot under that hair and its base. There is also some discomfort in attaching the thing to your hair or scalp.
- Easy to spot. The sales pitch states you'll never notice a good one—it looks like the real thing. Baloney! While some are better than others, I've never been surprised by someone wearing this cover-up.

C. The Big Flap

Millions of men try to compensate for their baldness or thinning top by growing hair long on one side, then combing that excess hair over their sparse dome. This is effective advertising to anyone with the slightest hair-sense that the flap-wearer is "hiding in the closet" about a very natural phenomenon. To attempt this cover-up, you must **carefully** part the long hair on the lower side.

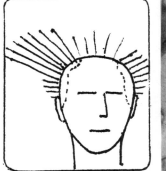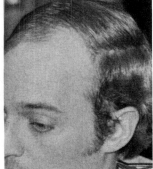

Some wear a few long strands over the top just for a laugh, but the big majority actually think they're pulling off some sort of deception. When the head is tilted forward or it's viewed from behind, that shiney scalp exposes their flim-flam. Normal top hair also has some fullness; the flap lies flat as a pancake on top. Long strands bunched together to resemble a front hairline is another sure sign.

This way of wearing hair has some negative health consequences:
- It needs a lot of time to get it to lie "just right" and more than a little time and concern to **keep** it that way throughout the day. A windy day is never a good day—mental health is bound to suffer.
- Besides being burdensome, the flap takes away from the growing health of the surviving hairs on top. Because of the long-haired flap's weight, a lot of bending occurs at the roots. You also have an untouchable creation that won't receive any blood flow stimulation like you get from a scalp massage, or even handcombing.

I give these haircuts from time to time, but only because I want to gain that fellow's trust so he might consider accepting his hairloss and my preferred way of dealing with it. (To hint at a new approach to a first-timer who has spent a good chunk of time and energy with the flap, is to—in most cases—**blow** him right out of the chair.)

D. A Healthy Way to Make the Most of What You Have

How people react to hairloss varies as much as night and day. Many cancer chemotherapy patients get so depressed over their unavoidable hairloss, they lose that fighting spirit so needed to be a survivor. On the other hand, I saw two women on an interview program: both had alopecia universalis (total loss of hair), and for a variety of reasons, both expressed a genuine sense of liberation because of their hairless condition. Many cling to their flaps and cover-ups as if the number of hairs on their heads was an important measure of their self-worth. Some feel hairloss just makes haircare easier.

From my experience, most fellows already practice or are willing to

* * *

Security depends not so much on what you have, as much as what you can do without.

                                                                    Anonymous

try this relaxed approach that meets hairloss head-on. Yes it takes some self-assurance and acceptance of reality, but even the timid can appreciate the carefree nature of it, plus the healthy benefits. The haircutting how-to depends on the kind of hairloss.

1. **Thinning hair**. When the hair is in any stage of thinning, you cut any of the three basic haircuts as if you were working on a full head of hair. The only difference is to cut the top hair a little shorter (1/2 - 1 inch) than usual. Doing this adds extra fullness and will cover most domes as well, and in many cases, better than the long-haired flap. Page 20 has examples of this shorter cutting.

As you can imagine, a receding hairline or bald spot won't be hidden by the extra fullness: this is where acceptance is needed.

2. **Total baldness on top**. When the top gets to the shiney stage and hairgrowth is limited to the horseshoe around the sides and back, you only need to follow the sequence of cuts for the sides and back with any of the three haircuts or their variations. If there are a few pesty stragglers on top, give them a shorter equal-length cutting or cut them off altogether by using the finger-bracing method close to the scalp, or they can even be shaved off.

11.12 HOME HAIRCUTTER'S SUPPLY

By the time this book is published, I will have set up a mail-order business that offers low to moderate priced haircutting tools of the highest quality. If given proper care, your grandchildren will be able to use these tools for their hair needs.

All the tools shown in the book will be offered, and each is fully guaranteed. Because of changing prices and new tools offered, an updated brochure will come out on January 1 of each year—to receive the current brochure, send a self-addressed, stamped, business-size envelope to: Home Haircutter's Supply, P.O. Box 11400, Minneapolis, Minnesota 55411

Any cutting tool eventually needs sharpening. I get by well with a once a year trip to my sharpening expert; you can expect to sharpen your tools every 5 years or more, depending on how much cutting you do. Home Haircutter's Supply will have expert tool sharpening and repair service for the tools we sell. Details are in the brochure.

11.13 HAIRCUT RECORDS

Keeping track of how you cut someone's hair is easily done if you use the method I've developed. I use a Polaroid camera to take a picture of the finished haircut, then write the particulars (kind of haircut, length it was left, problem areas, haircare suggestions, etc.,) at the bottom of the photo. With their name on top, it's filed in my index card file and I'm ready for their next visit. By doing this, I don't have to go through a second "question and answer" session as to their hair desires. This method is also valuable for making improvements on future haircuts: when they come back I ask how the last haircut was—if they want if left longer or cut shorter, or shaped a little different, knowing exactly what was done the first time makes it easy to modify the second cut to the changes they have in mind.

Maybe your memory is good enough to avoid this, buy I deal with too many people to try to keep this information in mind. On the other hand, even if you don't need the reminders written at the bottom of the photo, it's kind of nice to have a visual diary of your haircuts.

11.14 IN CLOSING

Writing a book isn't like anything I've attempted before: the time it takes and the difficulties involved are much more than I expected. A couple of writing goals kept me plugging away—slowly, but surely, I felt I was getting closer to these aims.

- De-mystify the subject of hair and its care: what it is, how it's easily and healthfully cared for, and how to give well-done haircuts.
- Contribute to a kind of freedom: helping people become a little more self-reliant, and showing what it takes to make hair ignorable throughout the day.

While on these last-minute ponderings, a plug for the **essential** you is in order. We're bombarded daily by slick sales pitches telling us happiness comes with a certain look, the latest thingumajig—you'll be O.K. if you buy. . . . As this relates to hair, inventive folks have come up with all manner of costly ways to change the natural state of those little thread-like objects. Why? How is it possible to improve on healthy, clean, well-cut hair that is a natural consequence of one's genetic heritage?

Going beyond the treatment of hair, I believe our world is a little better place when anyone chooses a lesser emphasis for the material side of their being, and instead, decides to put primary emphasis on their inner being. Selecting a simple, less-is-better approach to life that emphasizes health and harmony while avoiding outward ways of seeking self-worth, says a most positive thing about **WHO YOU ARE**.

I'll keep my fingers crossed that you freely give your haircutting skills to others. Your sharing will help get some good going around: what **YOU** send out travels a long ways, but it always comes back.

HAPPY HAIRCUTTING!

* * *

If we want to make something really superb of this planet, there is nothing whatever that can stop us.   Shepherd Mead

We have probed the earth, excavated it, burned it, ripped things from it, buried things in it, chopped down its forests, leveled its hills, muddied its waters and dirtied its air. That does not fit my definition of a good tenant. If we were here on a month-to-month basis, we would have been evicted long ago.

                    Rose Bird, Chief Justice of the California Supreme Court

The world is being run by (people) who really take no responsibility for future generations. And in this day and age, with science as it is, we have to be responsible or we won't survive.   Dr. Helen Caldicott

Technological progress has merely provided us with more efficient means for going backwards.   Aldous Huxley

Pollution is our most important product.   Message on Earth Day button

The world is composed of "takers" and "givers". The takers eat better, the givers sleep better.   Anonymous

We cannot hold a torch to light another's path without brightening our own.   Ben Sweetland

Life's arithmetic is funny; when you get to the end, what you have is what you have given away.   Anonymous

I expect to pass through life but once. If therefore, there be any kindness I can show, or any good thing I can do to any fellow being, let me do it now, and not defer or neglect it, as I shall not pass this way again.   William Penn

SUBJECT INDEX

CAN'T FIND IT? LOOK THROUGH
THE CONTENTS LISTING AT THE
BEGINNING OF THE CHAPTERS.

ACKNOWLEDGEMENTS

It is one thing to know how to cut hair and to teach others by demonstrating this skill. It is altogether something else to explain haircutting on the printed page. During the years I have worked on this project, I've had invaluable help from some special folks.

David Burke has taken my rough subjects and verbs and molded them into an understandable piece of reading; Dave has provided the main editing help and encouragement I needed. As the book was progressing my wife Nancy, daughter Kris, neice Alison, sister-in-law Pat, and good friend and fellow barber Randy Sievert were a big help in freeing the manuscript of those little, easy to overlook errors. In the final stages Elizabeth Knight proved to be the wordsmith this book needed.

Lenny Hedahl has taken care of the bulk of the photography. His quality work gave real meaning to the notion of a picture being worth a thousand words. Tim Zniewski helped out on the early photos that allowed me to zero-in on the later, more accurate photos. Bonita Thurner and my nephew Kevin Smith advised me on my illustrating efforts. Another nephew, Toby Smith, designed the front cover.

Bettye Titus and my brother Dick did the word processing on the earlier drafts of the book. The typesetting was done at Stanton Publications Inc., with the help of Don Leeper and David Tripp. Armon Roshen of Viking Press Inc., steered me through the printing process. All contributed in significant ways.

With so many photos and illustrations, the book had many "white spaces" at the bottom of pages. The quotes of wit and widom used to fill those spaces came from the following sources with permission to reprint: The Mother Earth News magazine; Minneapolis Star and Tribune newspaper; Peter's Quotations: Ideas for Our Time by Dr. Laurence J. Peter (Wm. Morrow and Co. Inc., 1977); and from the soon-to-be-published Banter, Barbs and Brass Tacks by James H. Sowell. (Mr. Sowell's excellent collection is the source of most of the "anonymous" quotes found in the book—I would be grateful to hear from anyone who can shed light on the authors of those quotes so credit can be given in future printings.)

Moral support, when it seemed I had taken on more than I could handle, came from many: my wife and children have been extra special in their help and sacrifices. Friends Rick Bennett, Tom Ennen, Jeanette and Jerry Fair, Craig Luedeman, Mary Robishon, Don and Sue St. Dennis, Ginny and Ralph Witcoff—they were buddies when I needed them and understanding when I wasn't available.

I owe special thanks to my parents. Mom and dad's unselfish aid came in many forms, and was largely responsible for me having the time to spend on this project—without their help I couldn't have done it. Dad's tips, explanations and demonstrations gave me a solid foundation for my haircutting career—his pearls of wisdom have proven to be right on the mark over and over again.

Thanks to my customers. You endured my erratic work hours and too much talk about this project. Your encouragement and financial support helped to bring this project to completion.

Last, I want to thank you for buying the book—I hope you found it a good investment of money and time. Just as you'll want to make improvements on your beginning haircuts, so I want to do all I can to improve this book. Future editions of the book will have changes based on the kind of feedback I get from my readers—I'll appreciate any comments, suggestions, criticisms, etc., you care to make.